77
Outrageously Effective Anti-Aging Tips & Secrets

Natural Anti-Aging Strategies & Longevity Secrets Proven to Reverse the Aging Process

+ 30 Outrageously Awesome Natural Beauty Tips

Amy Waldow

ISBN-13: 978-1469997544
ISBN-10: 1469997541

First Printing, 2012

Printed in the United States of America

Disclaimer and/or Legal Notices

The information contained herein reflect the opinions and up-to-date research of the author and is believed to be accurate and sound, but should not be construed as personal medical advice, diagnosis, or treatment. It is intended to provide helpful, educational, and informative information on the addressed subjects. Specific medical advice and instruction should be obtained from a licensed health care practitioner.

The author and publisher are not responsible for any adverse reactions that may result from the use of suggestions or preparations discussed in this book, and do not accept liability for those who choose to self-prescribe.

Always consult with your doctor or a health professional before beginning any diet, nutrition, lifestyle, exercise, or weight loss program.

Liability Disclaimer

By reading this book, you assume all risks associated with using the advice given, with a full understanding that you, solely, are responsible for anything that may occur as a result of putting this information into action in any way, regardless of your interpretation of the advice.

You further agree that the author and/or publisher cannot be held responsible in any way for the success or failure, as a result of the information presented in this book.

Terms of Use

You are given a non-transferable, "personal use" license to this book, and are not allowed to distribute this book.

Also, there are no resale rights or private label rights granted when purchasing this book. This book is only for your own personal use.

77
Outrageously Effective Anti-Aging Tips & Secrets

Natural Anti-Aging Tips & Longevity Secrets Proven to Reverse the Aging Process

+ 30 Ourageously Awesome Natural Beauty Tips

Table of Contents

Author's Introduction:..11

Part I: 13
10 Anti-Aging Tips That Will Kick-Start Your Health and Immune System 13
1. Mastering Stress for Optimal Health 15
2. Practice Meditation for Inner Peace 19
3. PURE Water: The Ultimate Anti-Aging Tonic 21
4. Life-Extension Through Exercise 23
5. Discover the Healing Powers of Yoga, Qigong, & Pilates 27
6. Power Foods to Super Boost Your Immunity............37
7. All-Natural Vitamins & Supplements for Superior Health 45
8. Self-Massage: Bliss Through Self-Touch 49
9. Catch Up On Your Zzz's 53
10. End Adrenal Fatigue & Reclaim Your Energy 57

Part II: 61
12 Anti-Aging Tips That Help Prevent Premature Aging 61
11. Anti-Inflammatory Diet & Nutrition 63
12. Antioxidant Super Foods for Super Health & Disease Prevention..71
13. Middle Age Spread: Say Goodbye to Belly Fat 75
14. Tame the Sugar Beast...79
15. Stay Young: Consume More Healthy Fats 81
16. Probiotics: Friendly Bacteria for a Healthy Gut........87
17. Fiber: Get Smart About Digestive Health 91
18. Life-Extending Anti-Aging Herbs 93
19. Improve Brain Health & Performance 97
20. Break Unhealthy Bad Habits 101
21. Prevent Osteoporosis Through Diet & Lifestyle 103
22. Arthritis Prevention: Life Without Pain 107

Part III: 109
6 Anti-Aging Foods That Offer a Powerhouse of
Nutrition 109
  23. Hemp, Chia & Flax: Seeds of Life 111
  24. Extra-Virgin Olive Oil: A Powerful Age Reversing
      Elixir 117
  25. Acai Berry: Nature's Energy Fruit 121
  26. Aloe Vera: The Multi-Purpose Miracle Plant 123
  27. Apple Cider Vinegar: Harness it's Healing Powers
 127
  28. Green Tea: The Natural Healing Brew 131

Part IV: 133
5 Anti-Aging Tips That Work Like Magic 133
  29. Facial Exercise: The Natural Facelift 135
  30. Hydrotherapy: For Healthy, Youthful, Vibrant Eyes
 137
  31. DIY Scalp Massage: Relax & Stimulate 139
  32. Skin Needling: Anti-Aging Skin Rejuvenation
      Treatment 141
  33. Stop Thinning Hair and Hair Loss 145

Part V: 149
8 Anti-Aging Tips That Have a Profound Impact on
Your Health 149
  34. Diaphragmatic: The Correct Way to Breathe 151
  35. Dry Skin Brushing: Health & Beauty Treatment ...153
  36. Detoxify Your Body Naturally 155
  37. Sweat Your Way to Radiant Health 159
  38. Chew More, Eat Less, Live Longer 161
  39. Practice Emotional Freedom Technique
      (EFT Tapping) 163
  40. Oxygenate With a Chi Machine 165
  41. Color Therapy: Healing With Color 169

Part VI: 173
6 Tips That Will Make Your Libido Soar 173
  42. Eat a Libido Boosting Diet 175

43. Balance Your Hormones Naturally 177
44. Herbal Remedies to Restore Low Sex Drive 179
45. Kegel Exercises for Better Sex 183
46. Ignite Your Sex Life 185
47. Aromatherapy for Menopausal Relief 187

Part VII: 193
**10 Anti-Aging Tips That Have a Dramatic Impact on
Your Skin's Health** 193
48. Avoid Excessive Sun Exposure 197
49. Use Cutting Edge Skin Care 203
50. Exfoliate Your Way to Radiant Skin 209
51. Lighten & Brighten Your Skin 211
52. Beauty Serum: The Magic Skin Elixir 213
53. Mask Your Imperfections 215
54. Replenish Lost Moisture 217
55. Consistency with Skin Care is Key 219
56. Natural Homemade Skin Care Recipes 221
57. Diminish Cellulite Naturally 229

Part VIII: 233
**20 Anti-Aging Tips That Promote Peace, Harmony,
and Longevity** 233
58. Be True to Yourself 235
59. Create Balance in Your Life 237
60. Find Pleasure Daily 239
61. Make Self-Care a Top Priority 241
62. Listen to Your Body and Soul 243
63. Discover Your Life's Calling 245
64. Learn Something New Every Day 247
65. Arouse & Nurture Your Passions 249
66. Step Out of Your Comfort Zone 251
67. Adjust Your Attitude 253
68. Laugh Your Troubles Away 255
69. Make Friends and Be Social 257
70. Slow Down and Pay Attention............................259
71. Think Positive Thoughts 261
72. Keep the Focus On You 263

9

73. Live in the Present Moment 265
74. Let Go of Negative Emotions 267
75. Treasure Life's Simple Pleasures 269
76. Keep a Gratitude Journal 271
77. Celebrate Life and Find Magic in Every Day 273

In Review... 275
In Conclusion... 283

Part IX: 287
30 Outrageously Awesome Natural Beauty Tips.....287

Author's Introduction:

There's nothing wrong with growing older—unless of course you're doing it too rapidly. Aging is a natural and inevitable part of life. Many people fear growing old, but as long as you're proactive about your health and aging with grace, there are numerous benefits to aging.

With age comes wisdom, stability, and security. Generally one's priorities have shifted and fewer things are taken for granted. You don't sweat the small stuff so much anymore and precious time spent with family and friends is more tightly embraced.

Then there's the downside of aging—sometimes our bodies fail us. As we enter mid-life and into our golden years, our ability to fight off infection, as well as other health related problems diminish significantly, and conditions such as heart disease, high blood pressure, arthritis, diabetes, and obesity significantly increase.

Our longevity is controlled by the lifestyle choices and decisions we make each and every day. If you are aging prematurely, chances are it's because of an unhealthy lifestyle, bad habits, or both. Years of consuming a poorly balanced diet (low in nutrients and high in calories), along with lack of exercise, chronic stress, negative emotions, and environmental toxins all have a cumulative effect and contribute to our immune systems inability to fight illness and disease.

That's why it's so important to keep our health in the best possible shape ever, by incorporating powerful, anti-aging immune boosters into our everyday lifestyle. Optimal health isn't just about healthy eating and exercise;

it's about taking care of our physical, mental, emotional, and spiritual health.

Fortunately, the body is remarkably regenerative. We can significantly increase our life expectancy by improving our diet with immune boosting nutrients, exercising on a regular basis, reducing stress, and taking care of our emotional health and well-being.

Imagine, if you could turn the clock back naturally— without prescription drugs or cosmetics surgery. The good news is, by practicing natural anti-aging medicine, you really can live a longer, healthier, happier life—and absolutely age with grace. And it's not as hard as you think...

Part I:

10 Anti-Aging Tips That Will Kick-Start Your Health and Immune System

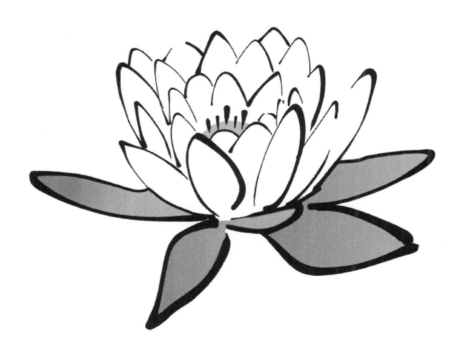

How fast we age and how long we live is largely determined by our immune system. The immune system is our body's natural defense system. While most of us take our immune system for granted (until we get sick), this remarkable and complex system is hard at work 24 hours a day, every day, fighting off foreign invaders like bacteria, germs, viruses, and toxins. These pesky invaders can weaken the immune system and cause everything from frequent colds, allergies, and premature aging to serious life threatening diseases such as cancer, heart disease, stroke, and diabetes.

Because our immune systems become less effective as we age, eating the right kinds of foods and living a healthy lifestyle is imperative for fighting off infection and disease prevention. Learning how to keep your immune system strong and healthy is the most important thing you can do to keep yourself disease-free and to help shield yourself from the many adverse effects of aging.

Implement These Powerful Steps to Slow Down the Natural Aging Process, Reduce Stress, Boost Your Energy Levels and Strengthen Your Immune System:

1. Mastering Stress for Optimal Health

Stress is one of the most serious health concerns in America today. Known as the "silent killer," stress (physical, mental, and emotional) causes us to age prematurely. Everyone has to deal with stress, whether it's stress from family, work, or from any other outside source. Stress is a normal part of everyday life, and some stresses actually prove beneficial—for instance, in a life or death situation. The problem is, when stress becomes excessive. Long-term chronic stress (stress exhaustion) not only makes you feel miserable, but it has a negative effect on your physical appearance—hair, skin, and your looks.

Stress Symptoms - Excessive stress takes an enormous toll on the immune system. High amounts of stress release hormones which depress the immune system and speeds up the aging process. Chronic stress is linked to physical, psychological, and emotional symptoms such as depression, irritability, frequent colds, headaches, heart disease, high blood pressure, digestive problems, sleep problems, obesity, and chronic disease.

Reduce Stress, Free Up Energy - If you truly want to slow down the aging process, incorporate anti-aging stress management strategies into your daily life. If you're experiencing stress symptoms, physical activity is a great way to blow off some steam. Check out a yoga class or spend time in nature. Or...

...Try These Other Healthy and Nurturing Stress Reduction Techniques to Help You Relax and Recharge:

Breathe - Good breathing equates to better health in all realms of life—physical, mental, emotional, cognitive, and spiritual. Sitting in a relaxed position, bring your attention to your breath. Inhale slowly and deeply through your nose, feeling your stomach expand. As you slowly exhale, gently pull your stomach in, making your exhalation twice as long as your inhalation. Do this for 5 minutes, or as often as needed when feeling stressed or cranky.

Meditate - Quiet your mind and relieve stress by practicing daily meditation. Whether you take a class or buy a video—learning how to meditate is a great way to find inner peace.

Soak in a Hot Bath - Light some candles, turn on some soft music, and sprinkle a few drops of essential oils in the water. Lavender works well for stress. Relax and breathe in the scent. Try to turn off negative thoughts and visualize a place or scenario that makes you feel good!

Massage - There is nothing like a good massage to melt away tension. If you don't have the time, or can't afford the luxury of having a professional massage—Do It Yourself! Starting at the head, use a small amount of warmed aromatherapy essential oil. Chamomile has a wonderfully calming effect. Massage the scalp with your fingertips and palms in a circular motion, working your way down the body. End with your feet, vigorously stimulating the pressure points.

Soak Up Some Sun - Many people experience mood dips, especially in the wintertime. 15-20 minutes of natural light a day, or even just 3-4 days a week, can have a dramatic effect on boosting your serotonin levels and can really boost your mood and spirit!

Take a Walk - Ride a bike, work out to an exercise video, make love, or do any activity that you enjoy! Just get your body moving and your blood flowing—30 minutes is all you need to help bring you out of the doldrums.

Dance - Burn off tension and lift your spirits with upbeat tunes that make you feel good. And sing! Even if you're no rock star... sing to your heart's content, as if you were!

Journal - Writing things down on paper can really help! Spend a few minutes analyzing your thoughts to determine if there are underlying thought patterns which may be causing distorted thinking. Maybe it's your memory cells that are negatively influencing the way you feel. Focus on thinking positive and try to let go of negative, self-destructive thought patterns. And make it a point to remember what you're thankful for.

Take your Supplements - In addition to eating a well-balanced diet, taking a good quality multi-vitamin with minerals and antioxidants is especially important in times of stress. Also, omega-3 essential fatty acids are essential (hence the name) for strengthening your immune system and combating stress.

De-Stress with Chocolate - Sometimes simple pleasures are the best. Go ahead, eat some chocolate. Chocolate is more than just a comfort food. Research shows that eating chocolate (primarily dark chocolate), reduces stress levels and has many health benefits. Packed with natural antioxidants, dark chocolate reduces blood pressure, cholesterol, and reduces inflammation that can lead to heart disease.

NOTE: If all else fails and you're still experiencing chronic stress symptoms, you may want to talk with a psychotherapist to help you deal with the issues that are causing you stress.

2. Practice Meditation for Inner Peace

Meditation is the art of silencing the mind through focus and breathing. The simple act of practicing meditation increases inner peace, while balancing your physical, mental, emotional, and spiritual state of mind. Practicing meditation daily has been proven to take years off your biological age by dramatically decreasing stress, anxiety, obsessive thoughts, and addictive traits, while relieving feelings of depression.

Meditation is a natural immune booster and has been shown to significantly reduce incidence of illness and disease, enhance memory, increase self-esteem, confidence, intelligence, creativity, and cognitive skills. When you meditate you produce pleasurable chemicals and hormones which make you feel blissful and happy. Start off with just 5-10 minutes a day and gradually work up to 40-60 minutes. The simple practice of daily meditation has been shown to not only have a huge impact on our health, but on our skin's health, as well.

Meditation for Over-Thinkers - We live in such a hectic fast-paced society, that it's created an epidemic of over-thinkers. Over-thinkers have a hard time turning off their minds. They are compelled to analyze and re-examine their thoughts repeatedly. When over-thinking becomes obsessive, it can be detrimental to your health.

What is Mindfulness Meditation? Mindfulness is a type of meditation that involves paying attention, being aware of your thoughts and actions, and being fully present in the moment. Our natural tendency is to stray from the "here and now," to past or future events, or to other issues or distractions.

The Power of Mindfulness - Mindfulness meditation brings about calmness and clarity for dealing with the pressures of everyday life. Mindfulness meditation has been found to help reduce and overcome addictive or self-destructive behavior patterns—and can be a very powerful tool for those suffering from over-thinking, as it can help unclutter the mind and constant noise going on in the head. When you begin practicing mindfulness, you should notice drastic improvements in how you feel about yourself, your relationships, and life in general.

What's the Difference Between Transcendental and Mindfulness Meditation? - There are many forms of meditation with many goals. Mindfulness meditation can be learned from a book, an online course, through meditation DVD's, or learned from a therapist; whereas transcendental meditation is based on a mantra (chanting) meditation and requires taking a 10-12 hour course taught by a certified instructor.

Bottom Line: Transcendental meditation is considered by many to be the most effective and beneficial meditation technique. While both of these forms of meditation differ considerably, they both produce relaxation and many of the same benefits such as stress reduction, self-healing, centeredness, greater awareness, inner peace, and spiritual growth.

3. PURE Water: The Ultimate Anti-Aging Tonic

Roughly two-thirds of our body weight is water. The amount of water in the human body depends on age, gender, and body fat percentage. Drinking water in its purest form is vital to overall health. Water not only hydrates—it helps cleanse and detoxify the body, aids in proper elimination, regulates body temperature, protects the joints and organs, and carries oxygen and nutrients through the bloodstream for optimal cell function. Every system in the body is dependent on water.

Dehydration Epidemic - It's estimated that roughly 75% of Americans are chronically dehydrated and don't even know it. The average person loses roughly 10-15 cups (3-4 liters) of water a day. We lose water through normal bodily functions such as breathing, perspiring, digestion, and elimination. For the body to function properly, we need to replenish this water through the foods and beverages we consume.

Toxic Overload - When you're dehydrated, it increases the concentration of toxins in the body which can lead to a host of symptoms, everything from chronic fatigue to premature aging. If you are thirsty, it means you're already dehydrated. Monitor your urine. A hydrated body should produce clear, colorless urine.

Drink Water First Thing in The Morning - After a long night's sleep, our body's are not only dehydrated, but contain higher levels of toxins. So, before you reach for your morning cup of coffee, drink an 8 oz. glass of water first.

Anti-Aging Colon Health - It's estimated that older people are five times more likely to develop constipation than younger people. Water is very important component for keeping your colon healthy and for avoiding constipation. Also, if you want to keep your skin smooth, supple, and radiant—water is the secret for maintaining healthy, younger looking skin.

Say NO to BPA! Our health is dependent on the quality and quantity of water we drink. Rather than buying bottled water which can contain harmful chemicals like BPA (Bisphenol A), instead, invest in a good water purification system, or opt for BPA Free clear bottles containing fresh purified, or spring water. Never use cloudy bottles!

Distilled Water: Healthy or Not? Distillation is the process in which water is boiled (to remove impurities), then evaporated, and finally the vapor (or steam) is cooled, condensed, and turned back into water. Drinking distilled water can leave you mineral deficient and your body highly acidic. Prolonged use and chronic acidity can lead to serious health problems, low energy levels, inflammation, and accelerated aging.

For Adequate Hydration - It's recommended to drink one half of your body weight in ounces per day. For example: a woman weighing 150 lbs., should drink 75 oz. of water per day. **NOTE:** Because obesity decreases the water percentage in the body, an overweight person needs one additional glass of water for every 25 lbs. of extra weight.

4. Life-Extension Through Exercise

Physical exercise at all stages of life is important; however, as we grow older many people instead, shy away from physical activities and become more sedentary. This is the time to really consider not only the physical and mental benefits from regular exercise, but the healing side to physical activity, as well. Regular, moderate, daily exercise not only improves our cardiovascular health, but it strengthens the immune system, while stimulating the lymphatic system..

Is Your Lymphatic System Clogged? The lymphatic system is one of the most important, yet often the most neglected system in the human body. The lymphatic system nourishes tissues and cells, while cleansing the body of toxins and waste. Unlike blood that is pumped by the heart, lymph is dependent on physical movement and exercise to circulate around the body. Stimulation of lymph flow is critical in preventing illness and disease. The more we move, the more waste is flushed out of our system. The less we move, the more toxins and waste build up and are stored in the body, which then become stagnant, and can lead to multiple health problems.

In Addition... As we age, we begin to lose strength, flexibility, and cardiovascular (aerobic endurance) fitness. Our bone density also decreases, as does our stamina, coordination, and balance.

Add Weights - While strength training is beneficial for people of all ages, it can be an especially beneficial component in slowing down the aging process. Strength training helps the body build and maintain lean body mass, increases bone density, boosts metabolic rate and energy levels, and relieves arthritic symptoms. Strength training done regularly, not only builds bone and muscle, but counteracts the weakness and frailty that's usually associated with aging.

NOTE: Be sure to ask for guidance before starting any strength training program, and check with your doctor before you start lifting weights if you have any medical conditions, injuries, or illnesses.

Stretch - Stretching is an extremely important aspect of exercising, and the anti-aging benefits from stretching on a regular basis, are priceless. When you incorporate stretching into your daily workout routine, it helps prevent injury to joints, tendons, and muscles, while improving flexibility and sense of balance. Stretching before and after your workouts will help you gain agility, so you will be more mobile and suffer from less pain associated with aging and stiff body parts.

Avoid Physical Limitations - By stretching, performing cardiovascular exercises, and strength training on a regular basis, this will help you avoid the physical limitations that many people experience as they grow older. Even if you've never exercised before, it's never too late to begin reaping the benefits that an active lifestyle has to offer.

Get Yourself Moving - Exercise is probably the simplest stress reliever available and is vital to health and happiness. Whether you take an exercise class, a 30 minute walk, go for a bike ride, or a swim—exercise elevates your endorphin levels and is a powerful tool in enhancing your physical, mental, and emotional well-being.

How Much Exercise and How Often? Fitness experts recommend getting your heart rate up a minimum of 3 x's a week for at least 30 minutes; and to get in a minimum of 2 - 15 minute sessions (30 minutes a week) of strength training. **NOTE:** You gain the most benefits from exercise, and reduce the risks, when you workout within your target heart rate zone. For most healthy people, it's recommended to keep your exercise target heart rate in the range of 60%-80% of your maximum heart rate.

Calculate Your Heart Rate - A simple way to calculate your targeted exercising heart rate: 220 – (your age) = maximum heart rate. For example: A 50 year old womans targeted exercising heart rate should be approximately 170 beats per minute.

Best Time to Exercise - While it's not mandatory to exercise first thing in the morning, there are plenty of health benefits. Early morning exercise jump starts your metabolism and keeps it elevated for hours, while accelerating the body's ability to burn more calories—resulting in the extra added bonus of fat and weight loss. An early morning workout gets it out of the way, and puts you in a healthy mind-set for the day ahead. It's estimated that roughly 90% of people who exercise in the morning, stick with it and stay consistent.

To Eat or Not to Eat? While there is some disagreement in the fitness community about whether to exercise on an empty stomach or not, many experts agree it's best to have a light meal (200-300 calories) containing carbohydrates and protein, such as a protein shake about 45 minutes before working out.

NOTE: If you can't fit in an early morning workout, don't worry... as long as you are exercising, you are doing yourself a great service, and getting numerous health benefits, no matter what time of the day.

5. Discover the Healing Powers of Yoga, Qigong, & Pilates

a) Yoga

While the word "yoga" may conjure up images of people sitting on floor mats twisted in pretzel shape positions, this Ancient anti-aging practice is much more than just stretching, sweating, and breathing deeply. Yoga, which originated in India, is a combination of exercise and meditation and has been practiced in Eastern cultures for over 5,000 years. The word yoga means to bring together or unite, as in the mind, body, and spirit. The physical, mental, and therapeutic benefits of yoga are numerous!

The Physical and Anti-Aging Benefits of Yoga:

- Enhanced Energy and Endurance

- Develops Balance and Coordination

- Promotes Cardiovascular & Circulatory Health

- Improves Flexibility

- Increases Muscle and Joint Lubrication

- Strengthens, Tones, and Builds Muscles

- Strengthens your Core

- Helps with Pain Management

- Accelerates Body Detoxification

- Improves Digestion and Elimination

- Improves and Corrects Posture

- Massages Internal Organs and Glands

- Lowers Blood Pressure

- Improves Sleep Quality

- Boosts Immune System

- Boosts Sexual Health and Intensifies Orgasms

- Promotes a Strong Lymphatic System

- Improves Metabolism Function

- Enhances Weight Loss

The Mental and Spiritual Benefits of Yoga:

- Increases Body Awareness

- Relieves Chronic Stress

- Relaxes the Body and Mind

- Teaches you to Quiet your Mind

- Teaches you to Live in the Moment

- Increases Self Knowledge

- Sharpens Concentration and Memory

- Helps you Feel at Peace with Yourself

- Helps you Discover your Life Purpose, Meaning, and Direction

- Helps you Age Gracefully

- Helps You Find a Deeper Spiritual Connection with Your Higher Power

The Most Common Hatha Yoga Styles Include:

ASHTANGA: *Power*

Ashtanga is the most vigorous and fast paced style of yoga and is the preferred choice of athletes. Ashtanga yoga does little meditation, but strongly emphasizes building strength, stamina, and flexibility. **Best For:** Ashtanga yoga is for people who are in good to excellent physical condition.

BIKRAM: *Heat*

Bikram yoga is generally referred to as "Hot Yoga" and is quickly rising in popularity. Bikram is practiced in a room heated from 100 to 110 degrees, which allows for loosening tight muscles, while the heat causes profuse sweating, which helps to detoxify the body. The Bikram method is a set of 26 poses that are performed in a standard sequence for 90 minutes. **Best For:** While the Bikram practice is considered an intense workout and may seem a little overwhelming to begin with, bikram is believed to be a powerful and effective, natural health treatment for people with chronic diseases and medical conditions such as hepatitis-c, diabetes, heart disease, high blood pressure, fibromyalgia, and arthritis.

IYENGAR: *Alignment*

Iyengar yoga is most concerned with body alignment, and holding poses over long periods. Iyengar uses props such as chairs, yoga blankets, blocks, straps, and pillows, in order to bring the body into alignment. **Best For:** Iyengar yoga is perfect for beginners and those who haven't exercised in a while.

KUNDALINI: *Awakening*

Kundalini yoga emphasizes breath in conjunction with physical movement. Kundalini yoga is designed to free energy from the lower body through breath, poses, chanting, and meditation. This allows the energy to move upwards. Kundalini uses fast, repetitive movements, rather than holding poses for a long time. **Best For:** Kundalini is considered a holistic form of yoga and is suitable for all fitness levels.

SIVANANDA: *Healthy Lifestyle*

Sivananda yoga emphasizes yogic breathing, physical postures, deep relaxation, and meditation. **Best For:** Sivananda yoga is a less athletic, gentler style of yoga and may appeal to someone looking for a more holistic form of yoga.

Sivananda Yoga Integrates (5) Lifestyles:

- Proper Exercise

- Proper Breathing

- Proper Diet

- Proper Relaxation

- Positive Thinking and Meditation

VINIYOGA: *Gentle Flow*

This slower paced yoga is a more individualized form of yoga. By practicing yoga postures, along with yogic breathing, Viniyoga develops strength, balance, and healing. The length and intensity is adjusted to each person depending on their needs and capabilities. **Best For:** Viniyoga is ideal for beginners, senior citizens, and people with chronic pain or in rehabilitation.

Best Time to Practice Yoga - Since the stress hormone cortisol peaks in the morning, practicing yoga in the early morning hours can help keep you balanced. Also, practice a few yoga poses any time you're feeling stressed or frazzled to lower anxiety and blood pressure.

Key Point: Yoga works as an anti-aging therapy. It rejuvenates and revitalizes the mind, body, spirit, and soul. It keeps your body fit, your mind active, your skin glowing, and makes you feel younger and more alive!

b) Qigong -

Qigong (pronounced: chee gung) and sometimes spelled chi kung, dates back to over 5,000 years ago in China. Qi is the vital energy of the body, and gong is the practice of cultivating self-discipline and achievement. Qigong is a mind-body, self-healing practice that integrates gentle, graceful movements, physical postures, breathing techniques, and focused attention to enhance one's physical, spiritual, emotional, and mental health.

The Anti-Aging and Health Benefits of Qigong:

- Good for Managing and Losing Weight

- Improves Chronic Fatigue

- Improves Metabolism, Digestion, and Elimination

- Boosts the Immune System

- Stimulates the Lymph System

- Improves Circulation

- Retards the Aging Process

- Reduces Tension, Blocks, and Stagnant Energy

- Lubricates the Joints

- Soothes the Nervous System

- Balances Right and Left Brain Activity

- Promotes Pain Management

- Builds Confidence and Self-Esteem

- Promotes Over-All Sense of Well-Being

- Promotes Mental Alertness and Clarity

- Increases Sex Drive

- Builds Energy and Stamina

- Promotes Relaxation

- Provides Inner Awareness and a Sense of Calm

- Stress Reliever

- Increases Intelligence

- Develops Psychic Ability

- Develops Discipline

- Develops Flexibility

Key Point: Now, more than ever, people all around the world are practicing qigong. Practicing qigong daily is an excellent way to keep your mind and body fit and healthy.

c) Pilates -

Pilates (pronounced: puh-lah-teez) and originally called Contrology, is a therapeutic, body-conditioning series of exercises that are designed to tone, build strength, flexibility, balance, and inner awareness while realigning the body. Core stability exercises are a vital part of Pilates. The core muscles are the deep, internal muscles of the abdomen, back, pelvic floor and hips. When the core muscles are strong, they work together with the superficial muscles of the trunk. As you develop core strength, your posture will improve, and you will develop stability throughout your entire torso.

6 Pilates Principles - Essential Components in a Pilates Workout:

Centering - Physically Brings Focus to the Center of the Body (Powerhouse)

Concentration - Every Movement Requires Focused Thought and Direction

Flow - Exercises are Performed in a Continuous Flowing Graceful Manner

Control - All Exercises are Performed with Complete Muscular Control

Breath - Oxygenates the Entire Body while Cleansing it of Impurities

Precision - Every Exercise is Directed to Ensure Maximum Movement

Maintain Good Posture - As children we are taught to stand up straight, but as we get older many people have a tendency to slouch. Poor posture not only makes you appear older and more matronly, but over time may develop into the dreaded dowagers hump, a pot belly, a double chin, and a sway back. Poor posture also constricts your internal organs, giving them less space to function at peak efficiency. Poor posture can lead to chronic back pain and even make you lose inches from your height. Putting your body back in alignment will make you look slimmer, younger, and more attractive.

NOTE: Yoga, Pilates, and Qigong are all excellent for helping improve posture by strengthening, elongating, and aligning the spine and muscles that support the spine, while strengthening the core.

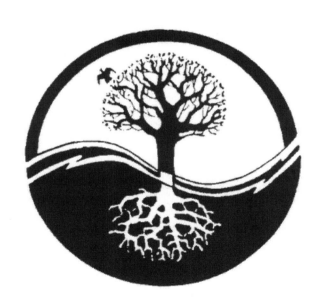

6. Power Foods to Super Boost Your Immunity

Nutritional, well-balanced eating is key in helping to strengthen the body's natural defense network. In order to keep the immune system functioning at peak performance—make the choice, to make good nutrition a top priority. It's vital for boosting energy levels and for overall health to include an array of colorful, antioxidant rich, high fiber, immune boosting, power-packed super foods in our diet every single day.

Go Organic - To help you maintain your health, eat more natural organic products. Many commercial products found on grocery store shelves contain chemicals, hormones, and other unnatural food additives which can trigger food allergies and compromise your health.

Alkaline vs. Acidic Foods - Every food and beverage we consume is either alkaline, acidic, or somewhere in between. Alkaline foods and acidic foods are measured in terms of pH (potential of hydrogen). A pH scale ranges from 0 (the most acidic) to 14 (the most alkaline). Ideally, the body's blood pH should be slightly more alkaline, ranging between 7.35 and 7.45 on the pH scale. The body has built-in mechanisms which keep it in balance. The problem begins when the body has to work over-time to keep it in balance.

Acid/Alkaline Imbalance - An imbalance in the pH level is commonly caused by eating too much acid-forming foods, as well as chronic stress. Excess levels of acid is often referred to as acidosis. The typical American diet is highly acidic. We consume too many foods and beverages like soft drinks, processed foods, junk food, fast foods, fried foods, refined sugar, high-fructose corn syrup, artificial sweeteners, etc.

When the body is in a chronic highly acidic state, it forces the body to rob vital minerals and nutrients from internal organs, muscles, and bones to neutralize the acid, leaving the body weakened. This can result in illness and chronic health conditions.

Most whole foods like fruits, vegetables, lentils, beans, nuts, seeds, and healthy fats are primarily alkaline. Whereas, foods like apple cider vinegar, lemons, and limes are acidic before digestion—the terms *acidic* and *alkaline* represent the effect it has on the body after digestion. These foods actually alkalize the body.

Are You Overly Acidic? A highly acidic body can cause a host of health problems. If you feel chronically tired, have low energy, poor digestion, food sensitives or allergies, and frequent headaches or colds—chances are you are overly acidic.

Other Health Concerns Resulting from High Acidity Include:

- Cardiovascular Damage

- Weakened Immune System

- High Blood Pressure

- Poor Digestion, Elimination & Flatulence

- Osteoporosis

- Obesity and Diabetes

- Osteoarthritis (Joint/Muscle Aches & Pain)

- Hormonal Imbalances

- Yeast and Fungal Overgrowth

- Various Forms of Cancer

- Skin Conditions (Rosacea, Eczema, Psoriasis)

- Accelerated Aging

Balance is Key - Experts recommend that ideally you should aim for a 70/30 ratio. Consume between 60-80% alkaline foods and no more than 20-40% acidic foods at each meal to restore pH balance in the body. The best way to balance the body's pH is by consuming a healthy nutrient-rich diet, getting proper rest, and limiting stress.

NOTE: If you want renewed energy, a leaner trimmer body, greater mental clarity, and overall health—you can simply go online and download or print out an Acid/Alkaline pH Food Chart which will show you which foods to eat in abundance, in moderation, and foods to limit or avoid altogether.

Low Glycemic vs. High Glycemic - Not all carbo-hydrates are created equal. Opt for low glycemic foods (complex carbohydrates) which release glucose (blood sugar) slowly and steadily into the bloodstream vs. high glycemic foods (simple or refined carbohydrates), which make glucose levels spike and are linked to health issues such as obesity, heart disease, and diabetes. It's vital for optimal health to include smart carbs like fruits and vegetables, which are high in fiber and water as your main source of carbohydrates. **NOTE:** Alkaline foods are usually low glycemic foods.

High Glycemic Foods to Limit or Avoid - Foods like white flour, white rice, white pasta, white bread, and low fiber cereals. Also, high sugar foods like cakes, cookies, candy, and soft-drinks.

Instead... Choose healthy low glycemic foods that can improve or reduce the risk of serious diseases from the list of healthy super foods below...

Powerful, Nutrient-Dense Super Foods That Will Strengthen Your Immune System and Can Add Years To Your Life:

Allium Family - Garlic, onion, shallots and leeks all help to detoxify the body and restore liver function and health, and are at the top of the list of foods that help prevent cancer.

Lentils & Beans - Low in calories and fat, but packed full of protein—lentils and beans are high in complex carbo-hydrates, fiber, folic acid, and both omega-3 and omega-6 fatty acids, and are an anti-aging dietary necessity.

Berries - When it comes to fresh fruit, berries are the richest source of powerful, anti-aging antioxidants, vitamins, minerals, and essential fatty acids (EFA's). The phytonutrients found in berries help discourage the growth of cancer cells, and the high vitamin-C content helps lower the risk of heart disease.

Cruciferous Vegetables - Broccoli, cauliflower, kale, cabbage, brussel sprouts, turnips, and bok choy are considered super veggies containing phytochemicals that have excellent cancer fighting properties.

Green Foods - Barley grass, wheat grass, spirulina, and blue green algae are all extremely anti-aging, and are shown to have beneficial effects on cholesterol, blood pressure, and cancer prevention.

Nuts & Seeds - Almonds, walnuts, cashews, and pumpkin seeds are tremendously nutritious and an excellent source of protein, potassium, fiber, and essential fatty acids. Nuts have numerous anti-aging and beauty benefits. **One Caveat:** Consume nuts in moderation if you're trying to cut calories as they are high in fat.

Omega-3 Fatty Acids - These "good fats" are found in foods such as salmon and tuna, flax seed (oil), hemp oil, avocado, and nuts. Omega-3 fats are essential for brain, cardiovascular, and skin health.

Soy - Tofu, soy, tempeh, and miso contain powerful cancer-fighting compounds known as isoflavones. Isoflavones possess active antioxidant properties, as well as antifungal and antimicrobial components which lower bad cholesterol, encourage bone density, and help reduce night sweats and hot flashes in postmenopausal women. **NOTE:** Because soy mimics estrogen, women who have, or have had breast cancer should consult their doctor about whether to include soy in their diet.

41

Spices - Used for centuries for their medicinal, as well as culinary purposes—cinnamon, turmeric, ginger, paprika, rosemary, cayenne, oregano, and basil actually have more disease fighting antioxidants than most fruits and vegetables.

Sprouts - Sprouts are one of the most nutritious foods that exists! They're extremely high in protein, vitamins, minerals, and antioxidants and have a high enzyme content, making them easy to digest. Sprouts are best eaten raw, as cooking destroys much of their nutritional content.

Yogurt & Kefir - Containing live cultures, these foods are vital for replenishing healthy flora in the digestive tract. Adding fermented (probiotic) foods to your daily diet will boost your immune system and increase your energy.

Whole Grains - Complex carbohydrates such as oatmeal, barley, brown rice, quinoa (keen wah), and popcorn are not only high in fiber, but a good source of vitamins, iron, and antioxidants. Whole grains have been shown to reduce the risk of heart disease, high blood pressure, and many types of cancer.

Say NO to Junk Food! Avoid excessive sugar intake, refined carbohydrates, processed foods, fast food, and junk food, as they've all been shown to weaken the immune system, lower your energy levels, and can lead to a host of health problems.

Retrain Your Taste Buds - Americans love fat, sugar, and salt because that's what we're used to eating. While it may seem foreign at first to eat mainly whole foods and a high fiber, plant-based diet—you can retrain your taste buds and learn to prefer a nutritious, clean, wholesome diet.

NOTE: And, while it's okay to eat a cheeseburger and french fries or donuts and ice cream on occasion—what matters most, is to make healthy eating a lifestyle pattern.

Key Point: If you're serious about preventing disease, boosting your immune system, increasing your energy levels, looking younger, and feeling your best—then learning to love anti-aging super foods is a must!

7. All-Natural Vitamins & Supplements for Superior Health

Along with eating a healthy diet, taking high potency anti-aging supplements are an excellent way to ensure your immune system is functioning at optimal level. Opt for a high-quality, multi-vitamin which contains a complete, balanced, nutritional formula that provides you with the essential vitamins, minerals, and potent antioxidants you need for optimal health and maximum longevity.

Our digestive system works hand and hand with our immune system, so it's important to also take a good probiotic to restore friendly bacteria.

Anti-Aging Nutritional Supplements That Help Turn Back the Clock:

Acetyl l-carnitine - This anti-aging brain nutrient helps prevent and increase brain receptors that would otherwise deteriorate with age. Effects include enhanced cognitive ability and a lessening of depression.

Alpha lipoic acid - Hailed as the most powerful antioxidant known to man—alpha lipoic acid is about 400 times stronger than vitamin-C, and may be the most important antioxidant of all for protecting the brain from neurological decline seen with aging.

Antioxidants - The principal antioxidants vitamins A, C, and E, selenium, and beta-carotene are all effective in helping prevent heart disease, cancer, stroke, and a variety of other diseases associated with aging. Antioxidants prevent disease by destroying free radicals inside the body.

Boron - Crucial for supporting bones—boron is a trace mineral that protects against osteoporosis, while preserving joint health. Boron is also beneficial for improving brain function and cognitive performance.

Calcium - Essential for strong teeth and bones—to be effective, calcium needs to be taken with vitamin-D and magnesium. **NOTE:** Calcium and magnesium work together to prevent osteoporosis.

Coenzyme Q10 - CoQ10 has numerous health benefits—it strengthens the immune system, lowers blood pressure, prevents heart attacks, counters obesity, and slows aging.

Essential Fatty Acids - EFA's are vital for the immune system, brain function, circulatory health, skin health, and anti-aging benefits. Omega-3 and omega-6 have different effects—borage and evening primrose provide omega-6, while fish oils provide omega-3 essential fatty acids.

Digestive Enzymes - Our bodies produce natural enzymes. When we're young we have an abundant supply, but as we age, we produce less. Many people think that taking digestive enzyme supplements are just for people with digestive problems—they are important for people of all ages—and they're especially vital as we age.

In Addition... Digestive enzymes are natural energizers that help us digest foods more completely. These enzymes are essential for the breakdown and absorption of nutrients needed for health and longevity. When foods are not digested properly, this results in a build-up of toxins and waste in the colon, which can result in digestive problems such as heartburn, constipation, bloating, gas, fatigue, and even bad breath. Using digestive enzymes assists in fighting aging by helping clean the colon, detoxifying the body, strengthening the immune system, and eliminating potential health issues.

DHEA - Is a natural hormone found in our body and produced by our adrenal glands. As we age, the levels decrease. DHEA can help with chronic fatigue, impaired immunity, heart disease, senility, and sexual dysfunction. DHEA is also known to lower the risk of cancer.

Phosphatidyl Choline - The main component of lecithin and needed for proper mental function—phosphatidyl choline helps prevent heart disease, gallstones, and liver problems, and has been found to be beneficial for neurological problems, memory loss, and depression.

Resveratrol (rez-VER-a-trawl) - This red wine extract is becoming one of the most talked about longevity products on the market today. Resveratrol is a powerful anti-aging antioxidant which lowers bad (LDL) cholesterol, while boosting your energy levels.

SAMe - Touted as an anti-aging, health-enhancing blockbuster—SAMe maintains mitochondrial function (the power generator of our cells) and prevents DNA mutations. In addition, SAMe protects the liver and heart and helps counteract depression.

NOTE: Unfortunately, studies show that many people are not getting the proper vitamins and nutrients they need to battle the aging process. While aging is inevitable—with the proper diet, exercise, and supplements, you can live a longer, healthier, more youthful life!

8. Self-Massage: Bliss Through Self-Touch

Daily self-massage is one of the easiest, yet most beneficial ways to maintain good health and well-being. Massage not only relaxes tired muscles, but it strengthens the immune system, improves circulation, aids in digestion, speeds up elimination of waste products, lifts endorphin levels, reduces stress, relieves tension, and promotes longevity.

Facial Massage - Over time, scrunching your facial muscles can lead to wrinkles. Regular massage of the facial muscles is not only extremely relaxing and a great way to unwind, but can help soften fine lines and wrinkles. In addition, regular facial massage has been shown to improve circulation, release toxins, break down fatty deposits, and brighten the complexion—leaving the skin feeling softer, smoother, and more vibrant.

Massage Your Entire Body - Start with the scalp, ears, face, and neck—move on to the shoulders, arms, and hands—and then to the front and back of the torso, ending with the legs and feet. These are the very basic self-massage techniques, but there are books and websites dedicated to this very effective form of treatment—and all it takes is 10-15 minutes a day.

NOTE: When massaging bare skin, use massage oil for better glide and less friction.

Reflexology Foot Massage - For instant relaxation, target your feet. A good reflexology foot massage works with the thousands of nerve endings in the soles of your feet, and is incredibly healing to the entire body. By using acupressure massage techniques and applying pressure to certain pressure points on the feet that are associated with the body organs—this stimulates energy flow throughout the entire body—reducing stress, and improving overall health and well-being.

NOTE: A reflexology chart is a valuable resource and great visual aid for anyone interested in giving a good foot massage.

Tennis Ball Foot Massage - For tired, achy feet—pamper your feet with a rolling foot massage. Either standing or sitting down—place a tennis ball underneath the ball of your foot (always barefoot), and slowly roll it back and forth under the arch, heal, and toes several times. Cover the entire foot, using your weight to press down, and put steady pressure on any sore, or tender spots.

Reflexology Ear Massage – The ears (just like the feet) contain reflexology and pressure points. Ear reflexology has been used for centuries for health, healing, and stress relief. Use your thumbs and index fingers to rub and gently tug on the lobes. Rub all the curves and folds of each ear, including behind your ears. This not only feels really good, but it triggers the release of endorphins, and stimulates energy points that connect to the organs and run through the entire body.

Reap the Benefits - So, when it's not in your budget, or you can't find time to visit a Massage Therapist, you can still reap the many benefits of this age old healing practice, by using your own hands.

Self-Massage Techniques: The 5 Basic Massage Strokes Include:

- Effleurage (long, fluid, gliding)

- Petrissage (kneading, squeezing, compression)

- Friction (deep, circular rubbing)

- Tapotement (percussion, cupping, tapping)

- Vibration (very light, rapid shaking)

Massage Oils - Massaging your body parts with a few drops of aromatherapy essential oils** diluted with a carrier oil, will reduce friction and skin irritation, while helping you work your muscles deeply.

Just Remember... A massage should feel good. DO NOT press too hard! **NOTE:** For more information on aromatherapy essential oils and carrier oils—please refer to tip # 47.

**Aromatherapy Essential Oils - Aromatherapy has been used for therapeutic purposes for over 6,000 years. Aromatherapy is a form of alternative medicine that uses natural oils obtained from plants for the purpose of promoting health, healing, and wellness. Our sense of smell is one of our most powerful senses and is linked to the emotional center of the brain. By inhaling the aroma or applying it to the skin, essential oils have the power to transform our emotions and heal our physical bodies.

51

Foot Reflexology

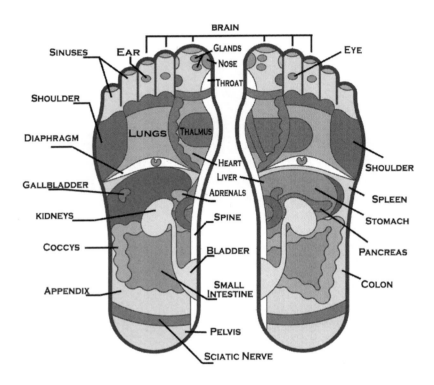

9. Catch Up On Your Zzz's

The importance of getting enough sleep cannot be over-stated. One-third of our life is spent sleeping. Sleep plays a vital role in promoting good physical health, longevity, and emotional well-being. Sleep consists of various stages and cycles that refresh and rejuvenate the mind and body.

Unfortunately, we live in a sleep deprived society, causing many people to experience fatigue, lethargy, moodiness, depression, poor memory, impaired motor skills, burnout, and stress.

Getting sufficient sleep is as important as a healthy diet and exercise. Our bodies go into repair mode while we sleep, replacing and rebuilding cells, muscle, and tissue, while boosting our immune system. The quality of our sleep affects the quality of our life including cognitive benefits, productivity, creativity, emotional balance, and physical vitality. Most healthy adults need between 7-9 hours of sleep a night to function at their best.

NOTE: Just remember though, that you can get too much of a good thing. Sleeping for more than 9 hours is associated with lowering energy levels and increased illness.

10 Tips to Help You Get a Good Night's Sleep:

1. Go to bed at the same time every night, even on the weekends. Your sleep cycle needs to have a regular rhythm.

2. Stay away from caffeine, nicotine, and alcohol for 4 hours before bed. Try sipping chamomile tea 30 minutes before bed, instead, to help wind down—or try 2 tsp. of apple cider vinegar mixed with 8 oz. of water, sweetened with a little honey. This healthy concoction right before bed, may work better than counting sheep. **NOTE:** For more information, as well as the many natural healing benefits of apple cider vinegar—please refer to tip # 27.

3. Avoid heavy meals or snacking for 2 hours before bed —but then again, don't go to bed too hungry, as that can interrupt your sleep, as well.

4. Do not exercise for at least 4 hours before bed. Exercising in the morning or afternoon is preferable, and will help to induce sleep at bedtime.

5. Only use your bed for sleep (and sex). Refrain from watching television, reading, working on the computer, or paying bills in bed.

6. Develop night-time rituals before bed, such as listening to calming music or drawing a hot bath (90 minutes before bed) and adding 15-20 drops of lavender aromatherapy essential oils. Also, massaging your temples, neck, and shoulders with a few drops of lavendar (or orange) essential oils can help with insomnia and works wonders for stress, anxiety, and nervous tension. Light stretching and deep breathing are other simple, yet powerful relaxation techniques that can help induce sleep and stress relief. **NOTE:** For more information, as well as the many health benefits of deep breathing—please refer to tip # 34.

7. Emotional Freedom Technique or (EFT) has been shown to be very helpful for insomnia and sleep difficulties. EFT is a very powerful healing technique which involves tapping in a certain sequence on various acupressure points of the body. EFT can help balance your body's energy system and resolve some of the stresses that are contributing to the insomnia. **NOTE:** For more information on the numerous physical and emotional benefits of Emotional Freedom Technique—please refer to tip # 39.

8. Make sure your bedroom is conducive to sleeping. Your sleep environment can have a profound impact on the quality of your sleep. Your bedroom should be decorated in cool, calming, restful tones—not bold, bright, energizing colors that stimulate. Make sure the room is dark, or wear a sleep mask—and if you're bothered by noise, wear earplugs. Also, a cooler room is recommended. If your room temperature is too warm, it may be stuffy and uncomfortable. Also, make sure your room isn't cluttered or messy, as this can stimulate negative energy.

9. Throw away your old alarm clock. No one likes to wake up to the sound of a loud, shrieking alarm clock. Instead, invest in one of the natural light, stress-free alarm clocks that are designed to awaken you naturally.

10. Don't bound out of bed in the morning. First, take a few deep breaths, then stretch to loosen up tight muscles and to get your blood circulating, then smile! Smiling first thing upon awakening starts your day off on the right foot and can set a positive tone for the whole day. Next, open your blinds to let some natural light in.

NOTE: The major causes of restless sleep are worry and an overactive mind. If you have too much on your mind, write down last minute concerns, so you won't rethink them over and over. If you can't fall asleep in the first 15-20 minutes of going to bed, climb out of bed, go into another room, and do something non-stimulating in low light. Once you feel drowsy, return to bed and try again. If all else fails, you may want to try natural herbal remedies such as melatonin and valerian root which may help to reduce insomnia.

Take a Power Nap - Power naps are the new term for what used to be referred to as "catnaps." Power naps are a great way to catch up on some sleep and to help you recharge. Keep the nap short, 20-30 minutes max. Any longer than that, it has the opposite effect—putting you into a deeper sleep and more groggy when you wake up. When you awaken after your nap, you should feel more alert, energized, and in better spirits.

10. End Adrenal Fatigue & Reclaim Your Energy

Do you feel tired (or exhausted), overstressed, and burned-out no matter how much sleep you get? You may be suffering from adrenal fatigue, also known as adrenal burnout syndrome or adrenal exhaustion. It's estimated that roughly 80% of Americans will suffer from adrenal fatigue at some point in their lives.

The adrenal glands secrete cortisol, adrenaline, and other stress hormones that kick into high gear during times of intense anxiety or physical stress. When stress continues over a prolonged period of time, the adrenal glands can deplete the body's hormone and energy reserves. Many people don't realize that stress not only makes us age faster, but has a significant negative impact on the entire body.

Common *Causes* of Adrenal Fatigue:

- Physical, Mental, and Emotional Stress

- Excessive Exercise

- Over Work

- Depression/Guilt

57

- Anger/Anxiety/Fear/Worry

- Toxic Overload

- Emotional Trauma

- Over-Indulgence in Stimulants—Coffee, Tobacco, Narcotics

Common *Symptoms* of Adrenal Fatigue:

- Fatigue/Lethargy

- Light-Headedness, Dizziness, or Fainting

- Low Immune Function

- Slow to Recover from Illness or Injury

- Getting Sick Frequently

- Feeling Cold Frequently

- Environmental or Food Allergies

- Poor Memory/Concentration (Brain Fog)

- Excessive Salt or Sugar Cravings

- Excessive Hunger

- Diarrhea and/or Constipation

- Menstrual Irregularities /PMS

- Sleep Deprivation

- Chronic Illness

- Irritability

- Weight Gain

- Hair Loss

- Insomnia

- Low Sex Drive

- Low Blood Sugar

- Low Blood Pressure

- Dry Skin

The Good News is... Simple anti-aging tweaks to your self-care regimen can work wonders to help boost your adrenal health!

Avoid Low Blood Sugar - Skipping meals is one of the worst things you can do, as it lowers your blood sugar and your metabolism. Instead, eat 5-6 small meals instead of 3 large ones, and eat protein with every meal.

Avoid Caffeine - Or at least drink it in moderation, or better yet, switch to antioxidant-rich green tea. Also, avoid energy drinks! Energy drinks contain multiple stimulants that give you an almost instantaneous, but temporary energy boost, followed by a "crash and burn" effect. In addition to caffeine, limit or avoid alcohol, processed foods, and tobacco.

Pump Up Your Vitamins - Especially antioxidants like vitamin-C and B5, which are critical for adrenal health, and take a multi-vitamin for nutritional support.

Aromatherapy For Adrenal Support - Aromatherapy essential oils, diluted with a carrier oil and applied to the skin, are commonly used to support adrenal function. Spruce, pine, cedar, peppermint, and citrus essential oils can provide support in regenerating over-tired adrenal glands.

Herbal Supplements - Known as adaptogens—herbal supplements have been shown to help boost our ability to deal with stress. Ginseng, astragalus, cordyceps, licorice root, and rhodiola have been found to reduce fatigue, and decrease chronic stress associated with adrenal imbalance.

Lifestyle Modification - Managing and reducing overall stress is key! Incorporate walking, stretching, and relaxation techniques such as yoga, deep breathing, and meditation into your daily routine.

NOTE: If you think you may suffer from adrenal fatigue, contact your doctor. Adrenal Fatigue can be diagnosed with a blood test known as the Adrenal Function Test (AFT) which indicates inadequate levels of adrenal hormones. Reducing adrenal fatigue syndrome and improving adrenal function is extremely important for optimal health.

Part II:

12 Anti-Aging Tips That Help Prevent Premature Aging

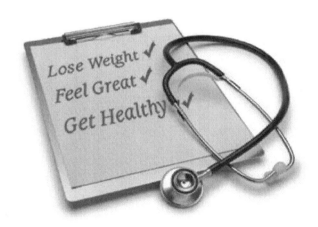

Americans are said to be the most self-medicated people on earth. We can rely on prescription drugs and surgery, or we can rely on our body to heal itself. And while prescription drugs and medication have their place, many alternative therapies can produce the same, if not better results, and without potentially harmful side effects.

We need to prevent disease through fighting off free radicals that can exacerbate premature aging. It's crucial to strengthen our immune system and rejuvenate our body with anti-aging nutrients to fight disease.

If you're not eating a healthy diet, and you're consuming too much highly processed junk food, it's bound to have a negative effect on your physical, mental, and emotional health. By over-indulging in a diet high in saturated fats, refined sugars and starches, empty calories, void of fiber, and low in antioxidants—this can have profound negative consequences on how you look and feel, as well as how you age.

The Following Anti-Aging Tips Will Help Restore Your Health and Vitality and Have You Looking and Feeling Fabulous in No Time:

11. Anti-Inflammatory Diet & Nutrition

Inflammation is an immune response by which the body's white blood cells protect us from infection and/or injury, and foreign substances such as viruses and bacteria. Most of the time this is considered a good thing, enabling our bodies to fight off various disease-causing bacteria, parasites, and viruses. The problem is, when it becomes chronic, inflammation destroys the balance in the body and can lead to a host of illnesses and diseases, which can play a key role in premature aging.

Chronic inflammation can slowly spread, speeding up the aging process, and causing chronic disease like heart disease, cancer, and Alzheimer's disease. Common symptoms of low-grade chronic inflammation are obesity, joint pain/stiffness, memory loss, congestion, acid reflux/heartburn, asthma, allergies, eczema, and even wrinkles.

The Good News is... Chronic inflammation can be reversed naturally through a healthy anti-inflammatory diet and by taking a high-quality multi-vitamin/mineral complex that provides powerful inflammation-cooling anti-oxidants like vitamins A, B, C, D, and E and selenium. Other inflammation-fighting dietary supplements include: fish or krill oil, CoQ10, and alpha lipoic acid, as well as herbs and spices such as ginger, turmeric, cinnamon, sage, oregano, basil, boswellia, and milk thistle.

Diseases and Health Conditions Linked to Chronic Inflammation:

- Acid Reflux/Heartburn

- Acne

- Aging of the Skin (wrinkles, loss of firmness)

- Allergies

- Alzheimer's Disease

- Arthritis

- Asthma

- Bronchitis

- Cancer

- Crohn's Disease

- Colitis

- Cirrhosis

- Dementia

- Depression

- Dermatitis

- Diabetes

- Emphysema

- Eczema

- Fibromyalgia

- Fungal Infections

- Gingivitis

- Heart Disease

- Hepatitis

- High Blood Pressure

- Insulin Resistance

- Joint Pain

- Metabolic Syndrome (Syndrome X)

- Obesity

- Osteoporosis

- Parkinson's Disease

- Periodontal Disease

- Psoriasis

- Sinusitis

- Tendonitis

- Vaginitis

Leading Causes of Chronic Inflammation:

Poor Diet - Consuming foods high in refined sugar, refined carbohydrates, high glycemic foods, processed meats, and especially foods containing trans-fats (hydrogenated oils) like fried foods, fast foods, and many processed convenience foods are often the cause of inflammation in the body.

Allergies - Chronic Food Allergies** or Food Sensitivities

Excess Weight - Obesity or Being Overweight

Stress - Chronic Psychological, Physical, and Emotional

Environmental Toxicity - Air, Water, & Food Pollutants

Bad Habits - Alcohol Abuse and Cigarette Smoking

A Sedentary Lifestyle - Little or No Exercise

How Do You Know if You Have Chronic Inflammation? There are tests you can take to determine the level of inflammation in your body, such as a C-reactive protein (CRP) blood test, as well as a fasting blood insulin test.

How Do You Reduce Inflammation in the Body? One of the easiest and most natural ways to reduce inflammation is to modify your diet and lifestyle choices. This means limiting or eliminating high-inflammation foods and adopting healthier, anti-inflammatory food choices, making exercise a priority, and if you smoke...QUIT!

What Kinds of Foods are Anti-Inflammatory?

Fruits and Vegetables - Brightly Colored Fruits and Vegetables (Preferably Organic)**

Good Proteins - Grass-Fed Lean Meats, Poultry, Seafood, Low-Fat Dairy Products, Beans, Legumes, Seeds, and Nuts

Omega-3 Essential Fatty Acids (EFA's) - Cold Water Oily Fish, Walnuts, Flax Seed, Hemp Seed, Chia Seed, Krill Oil

Healthy Fats - Extra Virgin Olive Oil, Flaxseed Oil, Hemp Seed Oil, Chia Seed Oil, Avocados, Nuts, and Seeds

Whole Grains - Whole Wheat, Brown Rice, Barley, Oats, Quinoa, Couscous

Whole Soy Foods - Soymilk, Edamame, Soy Nuts, Tofu,Tempeh

Herbs and Spices - Garlic, Ginger, Turmeric, Cinnamon, Rosemary, Basil, Cardamom, Parsley, Black Pepper

Teas - Green, White, and Oolong

Eat a Rainbow of Fruits and Veggies - It's crucial for good health, anti-aging, reducing inflammation, and disease prevention to include a wide array of healthy, vibrant colored seasonal fruits and vegetables in your daily diet. The deeper and brighter the color, the more vitamins and nutrients, as well as flavor are found in the produce.

There are thousands of health promoting phytonutrients (aka phytochemicals) found in brightly colored produce. Each of these food color categories (green, red/pink, orange/yellow, blue/purple, white/beige) contain different and unique phytonutrients which are essential to our health. Phytonutrients contain powerful antioxidant properties that protect the body against free radical damage and play a significant role in the prevention of disease and illness.

Green Fruits and Vegetables - Broccoli, zucchini, brussel sprouts, green peppers, green leafy lettuce, spinach, and kale protect the lungs, liver, arteries, and neutralizes carcinogens for cancer prevention, while promoting a healthy immune system.

Red/Pink Fruits and Vegetables - Tomatoes, red peppers, beets, cranberries, watermelon, and strawberries promote DNA and prostate health, lowers blood pressure and cholesterol levels, and helps in the prevention of cancer.

Orange/Yellow Fruits and Vegetables - Pumpkin, carrots, sweet potatoes, oranges, lemons, apricots, and papaya promote strong cellular communication, encourages alkaline balance, and supports good eye health.

Blue/Purple Fruits and Vegetables - Blueberries, blackberries, grapes, plums, eggplant, and red (purple) cabbage promote heart and brain health, supports healthy digestion, and fights inflammation.

White/Beige Fruits and Vegetables - Mushrooms, garlic, cauliflower, onion, and horseradish, as well as white flesh fruits like apples and pears promote healthy bones, cardiovascular health, balances hormone levels, lowers stoke incidence, and reduces the risk of cancer.

NOTE: Nutritional guidelines recommend consuming 5-9 servings of fruits and vegetables a day. And for the best all-around health benefits, make sure you're getting in at least 3 different colors of deeply colored fruits and vegetables. The more color variety in your diet, the better!

**Food Sensitivities - As we age, foods that never bothered us before, like dairy and wheat, may now trigger inflammation. A food sensitivity or food intolerance occurs when a person is unable to digest or break down certain foods properly. This can lead to chronic symptoms and illness.

Don't Ignore the Symptoms - It's important to listen to your body and identify your food intolerance(s). Symptoms may include diarrhea, nausea, gas, indigestion, stomach bloating or pain, headaches, tiredness, itchy skin, runny/stuffy nose, shortness of breath, and rashes.

NOTE: If you suspect you may have food sensitivities, keep a record for a couple of weeks of everything you eat, and any symptoms that may develop from specific foods. Then for the next couple of weeks, eliminate any foods that caused a reaction and see if the symptoms go away. If the symptoms persist, see your doctor or an allergist.

Key Point: Reversing and controlling inflammation is critical for optimal health and longevity. By reducing inflammation in your body, you'll not only look and feel younger, but you'll significantly lower your risk for chronic illness and disease!

12. Antioxidant Super Foods for Super Health & Disease Prevention

If you're not including powerful antioxidant-rich foods in your daily diet, then you're setting yourself up for premature aging, illness, and a variety of diseases. Antioxidants are a crucial component for eradicating free radicals.

What are Free Radicals? Free radicals are oxidants that break down healthy cells in the body. Free radicals are produced from everyday environmental toxins, as well as external sources such as stress, pollution, cigarette smoke, alcohol, excessive sun exposure, and pesticides. Foods high in antioxidants destroy free radicals that damage cells. Antioxidants also promote the growth of healthy cells and protects cells against premature aging, while strengthening the immune system and reducing the risk of diseases like cancer and heart disease.

The Most Common Antioxidants are: Vitamins-A, C, and E, beta carotene, selenium, and CoQ10. All-natural, anti-aging antioxidants are found in healthy high fiber fruits, vegetables, whole grains, nuts, seeds, and foods high in protein. If you really want to turn back the clock, while strengthening your immune system and reducing your risk of diseases like cancer and heart disease, add more anti-aging antioxidant rich foods to your diet.

Super Anti-Aging Foods High in Antioxidants:

Fruits - Blueberries, Strawberries, Cranberries, Raspberries, Acai Berries, Cherries, Red Grapes, Apples, Oranges, Grapefruit, Pomegranate, Papaya, Mangoes, Cantaloupe, Apricots, Plums

Vegetables - Carrots, Broccoli, Cauliflower, Cabbage, Sweet Potatoes, Tomatoes, Avocado, Asparagus, Beets, Artichokes, Peppers, Spinach, Kale, Pumpkin

Legumes - Lentils, Split Peas, Soy Beans, Kidney Beans, Black Beans, Pinto Beans

Nuts & Seeds - Sunflower Seeds, Pecans, Walnuts, Almonds, Brazil Nuts, Pistachios

Oils - Extra Virgin Olive, Walnut, Coconut, Flaxseed, Hemp seed, Chia Seed

Whole Grains - Oatmeal, Brown Rice, Wheat Germ, Brewer's Yeast, Buckwheat, Barley, Quinoa

Protein - Shell Fish, Tuna, Salmon, Chicken, Red Meat, Eggs, Cheese

Teas - Black, Green, White, Red

Spices and Herbs - Turmeric, Cinnamon, Ground Cloves, Oregano, Basil, Cumin, Parsley, Ginger, Sage, Dill Weed, Garlic, Onion

Occasional Indulgences - Antioxidants are also found in dark chocolate and red wine.

How Many Antioxidant Super Foods Should You Eat?
Nutritionists recommend getting in at least 5 servings a day. While that may seem high, it's really not, when you consider what counts as a serving: 1 cup raw leafy vegetables, 1/2 cup fruit or chopped vegetables, 3/4 cup fruit or vegetable juice, or 1/2 cup cooked beans.

NOTE: Antioxidants are also VITAL for skin health! Whether consumed through a healthy nutritious diet, supplements, or topical skin care products, antioxidants help reduce the signs of aging. Anti-wrinkle creams and skin care products containing antioxidant rich vitamin-C help to reduce fine lines and wrinkles, stimulate collagen and elastin production, and help to repair sun damage.

13. Middle Age Spread: Say Goodbye to Belly Fat

Obesity in the United States has become a major health issue in recent decades and is more prevalent than any other country. It's estimated that over 1/3 of American adults 20 years and over are overweight; another 1/3 of adults are obese; and nearly 6% are morbidly obese. That adds up to nearly 74% of American adults are overweight or obese. The average American gains from 1 to 1 1/2 lbs. per year after the age of 25. That's roughly 10-15 lbs. per decade. On average, obesity reduces life expectancy by two to four years, and morbid obesity reduces life expectancy by up to 10 years.

The Middle Age Spread - The "middle age spread" is the term frequently used to describe the extra weight gain that many men and women experience as they enter middle age. As we age, our metabolism slows down resulting in extra fat around our midsection. Combine that with a sedentary lifestyle and poor eating habits, and we're setting ourselves up for ill-health and premature death.

It's NOT a Big Fat Joke! Abdominal fat (visceral fat) is the deeply embedded fat that surrounds the internal organs. Visceral fat is different than subcutaneous fat, which is located underneath the skin. **NOTE:** For women, intra-abdominal fat has a tendency to become more prevalent, especially after menopause—this is the time,

75

when body fat tends to shift from the arms, legs, and hips, to the abdominal area.

Dangerous Fat - Weight in your midsection is more dangerous than the fat on your hips and thighs. Visceral is metabolically active fat that releases hormones and inflammatory substances into our systems that can be harmful to our health. Belly fat and obesity has been linked to adverse health conditions like diabetes, heart disease, cancer, high blood pressure, high cholesterol, high blood sugar, and stroke.

NOTE: If you're a woman and your waist is larger than 35 inches, or if you're a man and your waist is larger than 40 inches, reducing your belly fat should be a top priority!

How Healthy is Your Liver? The liver is an amazingly complex internal organ responsible for hundreds of functions in the body. The main functions of the liver is to filter toxins and wastes from the body, and produce bile, which helps to break down fats and food and convert it to energy. This remarkable organ also metabolizes proteins, fats, and carbohydrates, converts glucose into glycogen, produces certain proteins and cholesterol, and eliminates excess hormones.

Fatty Liver Disease: The Next Epidemic?? One-third of Americans suffer from a condition known as "fatty liver disease," also referred to as "non-alcoholic fatty liver disease." Unfortunately, many people are not even aware that they have it—and because you cannot see it or feel it —this chronic condition can go undetected for years. A fatty liver is the result of excess fat in the liver cells that replace healthy tissue—and is most commonly caused by obesity and a poor high-fat diet. The excess fat within the liver can lead to inflammation and affects it's ability to do its job well.

Does Your Liver Need to Go on a Diet? The good news is.. fatty liver disease can be reversible through gradual weight loss, by implementing a low trans-fat liver-friendly diet, and regular exercise.

Whittle Your Middle - The best way to lose belly fat and to cure fatty liver disease is through weight loss and a healthy lifestyle. Cut out, or reduce fatty foods, junk food, and fast food. Instead, consume a balanced, calorie and portion-controlled diet, rich in lean protein, fish, eggs, fruits, vegetables, whole grains, beans, seeds, nuts, legumes, and low-fat dairy products. Spreading your meals throughout the day, so you're eating 5-6 small meals a day is ideal for keeping your metabolism stoked. Combine a nutrient rich low-fat diet, along with both cardio exercises, that help you burn calories and fat, and strength training exercises, that help you build muscle, while reducing overall body fat.

Interval Training - Interval training is excellent for super-charging your fitness goals by revving up your metabolism, boosting your stamina, and burning off that excess fat.

What is Interval Training? Interval training is basically exercise which consists of sets of high intensity bursts of exercise for a short period of time, followed by low intensity exercise for a period of time. **NOTE:** Studies show interval training can produce incredible fat loss results in the belly, butt, and thighs.

Key Point: As you lose weight the healthy way, your body will reward you with increased energy levels, higher self-esteem, and a flatter belly, while reducing your risk of health problems.

14. Tame the Sugar Beast

The average American eats a whopping 175 lbs. of sugar a year. We all know sugar isn't good for us, yet it's become a key ingredient in the American diet. Sugar is basically just empty calories, void of any nutritional value, and depletes the body of vital nutrients. Yet, we love it, and it's become a rampant addiction.

Excessive amounts of sugar can lead to serious health problems including diabetes, heart disease, blood sugar imbalances, obesity, and premature aging. Consuming too much sugar also promotes inflammation in the body, and affects our mental health, leading to brain fog, depression, irritability, mood swings, panic attacks, and chronic fatigue.

What About High-Fructose Corn Syrup? High-fructose corn syrup (HFCS) is a highly refined man-made sweetener that's frequently used in place of sugar in tens of thousands of processed foods and beverages. Nutritionists have found HFCS to be a major culprit in our national obesity epidemic. Since HFCS was introduced in 1967 into the American food supply, obesity rates have skyrocketed. The corn industry claims that HFCS is perfectly safe when consumed in moderation—the problem is—Americans are consuming massive amounts.

Read Food Labels - Since high-fructose corn syrup is found in abundance in so many pre-packaged foods we eat, a good rule of thumb is to check food labels. If HFCS is listed as the first or second ingredient, consider purchasing something else.

Reduce Sugar Cravings - If you're one of the millions of people who are prone to sugar cravings, taking the supplement chromium picolinate may help. Chromium is an essential trace mineral that is found to reduce sugar cravings, while helping stabilize blood sugar levels.

Artificial Sweetener WARNING! In order to cut back on calories, many people have switched from real sugar to artificial sweeteners. These artificial sweeteners are used in abundance in almost every diet drink and reduced sugar product. The most popular artificial sweeteners are sucralose (Splenda), saccharine (Sweet 'N Low), and aspartame (Nutra Sweet and Equal). The problem is, artificial sweeteners are not good for you. Artificial sweeteners are man-made products made from chemicals that aren't meant to be ingested by the human body, and can cause a host of health problems.

Turn to Natural Sweeteners Instead - Honey, pure maple syrup, agave nectar, brown rice syrup, molasses, and stevia are just a few natural sweeteners that are actually healthy for you, and a good source of vitamins, minerals, and natural disease fighting antioxidants.

Indulge, But Don't Over Do It! While sugar is in no way considered to be a health food, it's a better option than high-fructose corn syrup or artificial sweeteners. So, if you'd like to indulge occasionally, go right ahead. Just treat your sugar-laden temptations as a treat, and NOT a staple in your daily diet.

15. Stay Young: Consume More Healthy Fats

Omega-3 (alpha-linolenic) and omega-6 (linoleic) fatty acids, also known as "essential fatty acids," are polyunsaturated fats that are essential for optimal health. Essential fatty acids (EFA's) are good fats that supply energy for the muscles, heart, and other organs. Since the body cannot make essential fats, you must get them through the foods you eat. However, it's vital to get your EFA's in balance, as high levels of omega-6's can actually block omega-3's health benefits.

Balancing Your EFA's is Key - While omega-6's are essential for good health, omega-6's tend to increase inflammation in the body; while on the other hand, omega-3's decrease inflammation. When the ration of omega-3's and omega-6's is out of balance, it not only accelerates the aging process, but the body may experience chronic inflammatory conditions that are linked to serious health conditions such as heart disease, stroke, cancer, obesity, diabetes, inflammatory bowel disease, Alzheimer's disease, Parkinson's disease, attention deficit hyperactivity disorder (ADHD), bi-polar disorder, and schizophrenia. A deficiency or imbalance of EFA's can also trigger autoimmune diseases like lupus and rheumatoid arthritis, and is a common cause of certain inflammatory skin diseases like eczema and psoriasis.

What About Omega-9 Fatty Acids? While omega-9 fatty acids are necessary and play an important role in health and disease prevention, omega-9's are not actually considered "essential" like omega-3's and 6's. Unlike omega-3 and omega-6 fatty acids, omega-9 fatty acids are a monounsaturated fat, naturally produced by the body, and are also found in many foods we eat. Olive oil (extra virgin and virgin) is one of the best sources of omega-9's, along with almonds, cashews, pistachios, pecans, macadamia nuts, avocado, and sesame oil.

NOTE: Many of the foods and oils we consume contain more than one type of fat.

Omega-3 Fatty Acids Reduce Inflammation in the Body and are Vital for:

- Brain Health (Cognitive and Memory)

- Cardiovascular Health

- Skin Health

- Joint Health

- Eye Health (Macular Degeneration, Glaucoma)

- Reproductive Health

- Immune Function

- Chronic Fatigue and Depression

- Type 2 Diabetes

- High Blood Pressure (Hypertension)

- High Cholesterol

- Reduction of Blood Clotting

- Osteoporosis

NOTE: It's best to consume omega-3 fats from the foods you eat, but for those who do not eat fish or foods containing omega-3 fatty acids, it's important to take a 500 mg omega-3 supplement daily.

Good Sources of Omega-3 Fatty Acids Include:

- Salmon

- Tuna

- Sardines

- Herring

- Mackerel

- Grass-Fed Meats

- Green Leafy Vegetables

- Whole Grains

- Legumes

- Beans

- Flax Seeds and Flax Seed Oil

- Hemp Seeds and Hemp Seed Oil

- Chia Seeds and Chia Seed Oils

- Krill Oil**

- Walnuts

- Hazelnuts

- Avocado

- Spirulina and Blue Green Algae

**Krill are small shrimp-like crustaceans found primarily in the Arctic and Antarctic waters. Krill oil is a superior source of omega-3's and is more than 50 times more potent than ordinary fish oil. And unlike fish oil, krill oil is loaded with natural antioxidants.

Avoid or Limit Refined Vegetable Oils - Sources of omega-6 fatty acids are found in extreme abundance in the typical American diet. Found in certain nuts and seeds—refined vegetable oils are routinely used in the majority of fast foods, processed snack foods, and sweets.

Good Sources of Omega-6 Fatty Acids Include:

- Eggs

- Poultry

- Grain-Fed Meats

- Nuts (Pistachios, Pine Nuts, Pecans, Almonds)

- Seeds (Sunflower, Pumpkin, Sesame)

- Chickpeas

- Whole Grains

- Cereals

- Corn Oil

- Canola Oil

- Safflower Oil

- Sunflower Seed Oil

- Evening Primrose Oil

- Borage Oil

- Pumpkin Oil

- Cottonseed Oil

Get the Proper Ratio - Most Americans consume very high levels of omega-6's and are deficient in omega-3's. The typical American diet consists of a ratio as high as 20:1 – 20 being omega 6's and 1 being omega-3's. This can spell trouble! The ratio to shoot for is 4:1 – 4 being omega-3's and 1 being omega 6's.

85

NOTE: It's important to emphasize, omega-6 fatty acids are not "bad," they just need to be consumed in the proper ratio.

Boost Omega-3's and Limit Omega-6's - To get your ratio to a healthy level, eat one or two servings of fatty fish per week along with whole grains, legumes/beans, nuts, seeds, and healthy oils—and cut your intake of fast foods and processed foods made with refined oils.

WARNING! It's important to eat moderate amounts of fatty fish. Fish is an excellent source of protein and loaded with vitamins and minerals and healthy omega-3's. But there is a downside to eating fish. Consuming too much fish can put you at risk of mercury exposure, which is a toxic substance. Certain kinds of fish contain more mercury than others—king mackerel, swordfish, shark, and tilefish contain the highest levels of mercury and should not be consumed at all, or at least eaten in very limited amounts.

It's All About Moderation - So, should you stop eating fish entirely? Absolutely not! But do eat fish in moderation. Opt for fish with low mercury levels like salmon, tilapia, chunk light tuna, whitefish, fresh-water trout, haddock, flounder, and shrimp.

16. Probiotics: Friendly Bacteria for a Healthy Gut

Probiotics are bacteria, also known as "good bacteria" or "friendly bacteria," that live in the body. There are literally trillions of both good and bad bacteria living in the human body. Most of these bacteria are not harmful, however, the gastrointestinal function may be affected when the bad bacteria, that make you sick, far outnumbers the good bacteria, that fight infection and kill bad bacteria. Stress, illness, and prescription antibiotics can throw our systems out of sync and deplete the body of good bacteria. Fortunately, probiotics can help to restore the "friendly bacteria, while maintaining digestive balance.

Probiotics for Antibiotics Side Effects - While antibiotics are typically prescribed to kill bad bacteria in the body, they also kill the good bacteria. To replenish the good bacteria, many experts recommend taking an acidophilis supplement (the most commonly used probiotic) and eating acidophilis-rich foods like yogurt and kefir daily for 2-4 weeks after the regimen of antibiotics is complete. **NOTE:** DO NOT take antibiotics simultaneously with probiotics, or they will cancel each other out. Overuse of antibiotics can lead to the creation of antibiotic-resistant bacteria, also known as "superbugs," making the antibiotics less effective, and has the potential of causing serious health problems.

When Ingested, Probiotics Actively Promote Overall Health in Many Ways:

- Stimulates the Immune System

- Reduces Negative Effects of Certain Antibiotics

- Promote Digestive Health

- Improves Absorption of Vitamins

- Inhibits the Growth of Harmful Bacteria

- Encourages Regularity

- Alleviates Constipation, Diarrhea, and IBS

- Reduces Lactose Intolerance

- Discourages Yeast Infections and Vaginitis

- Discourages Allergies and Asthma

- Reduces the Risk of Diabetes

- Reduces Inflammation

- Reduces Eczema Breakouts

- Promotes Healthy Skin

Add Fermented Foods - Yogurt and kefir contain live cultures that are vital for replenishing healthy flora in the digestive tract. Adding fermented (probiotic) foods to your daily diet will boost your immune system and increase your energy. For optimal health and well-being, take an acidophilus (probiotic) supplement to restore and balance your system.

Kombucha: An Ancient Probiotic Elixir - Kombucha (kom-BOO-cha) is a natural probiotic, that can best be described as a form of black or green tea, made of live bacteria and yeast, which has been fermented. Touted as a health elixir, this effervescent, tea-based beverage has been used for centuries for its many health, healing, and medicinal benefits, as well as a remedy for immortality.

Kombucha's Origin - Kombucha is traced back to China over 2,000 years ago, and it's popularity has since spread throughout the world. Kombucha has become very popular among celebrities and health-conscious consumers concerned with not only their health, but increased vitality, and longevity.

Kombucha's Health Benefits - Known for it's anti-aging, detoxifying, and energizing effects—the many health claims of kombucha include improvements and/or reductions in allergies, arthritis, blood pressure, cancer prevention, chronic fatigue, constipation, digestive health, hair loss and hair color restoration, immune strengthening, memory loss, metabolism enhancement, PMS, vision and eye health, skin health, and weight loss.

Does Kombucha Have Side Effects? While many people swear by its many health benefits, studies are inconclusive about the health claims of kombucha. Because kombucha has natural detoxifying effects, there have been reports of side effects such as stomach upset, nausea, vomiting, headaches, and diarrhea. These are common side effects that are often experienced in the first few days of detoxifying or cleansing the body. It's important to remember, that anytime you introduce something new to your system, you should do so gradually.

Kombucha's Recommended Dosage - If you are new to kombucha, start out with 2 oz. twice a day on an empty stomach, followed by a glass of water to flush out the toxins. Work your way up slowly to no more than 3 - 8 oz. servings a day maximum.

WARNING! Kombucha can be purchased commercially in stores, or can be brewed at home using a "kombucha starter kit." There are obvious safety issues involved in the at-home preparation and storage process to prevent contamination. The greatest dangers reported, came from those who consumed excessive quantities of kombucha, and from home-brewed kombucha that had been contaminated because of unsterilized conditions. **NOTE:** You should consult your doctor or holistic practitioner before taking kombucha, or starting any type of detoxification program.

17. Fiber: Get Smart About Digestive Health

Did you know that the average American eats just under 5 lbs. of food per day? That's roughly 1,500 lbs. of food per year and approximately 50 tons of food over a lifetime. That's a LOT of food we're consuming, and unfortunately, in many cases, up to 1/3 of this high food intake is junk food, void of adequate fiber and nutrition, and high in calories. With our crazy fast paced lives, many American's are just not getting enough fiber in their diets.

The average American now consumes less than half the recommended amount of fiber in their diet, consuming only 8-14 grams of fiber per day, while the experts recommend the daily allowance of fiber should be between 25-35 grams.

When you consume foods that are healthy for you, the nutrients are usually absorbed by the body. But fiber is different, it's not absorbed by the body—instead fiber is passed through the body undigested—therefore not absorbed into the bloodstream, but excreted from the body.

So, Why is Fiber So Important? Fiber, also known as roughage or bulk, is essential in our diets not only for digestive health, but in helping reduce the risk of some serious, chronic diseases. Fiber is a bulking agent that slows down the rate at which food enters the bloodstream, while increasing the speed at which food exits the body through the digestive tract. This keeps your blood sugar and cholesterol in balance, quickly eliminating harmful toxins from the body, and correcting digestive problems (which are epidemic today), thus reducing constipation, as well as other digestive health issues.

Natural Constipation Remedy - A low fiber diet, inadequate water intake, lack of physical activity, depression, and certain medications can all lead to chronic constipation. Good bowel function is vital for anti-aging health. Eating foods high in fiber not only helps you stay fuller longer, but keeps you regular, while boosting your colon health.

In Addition... Not only is fiber good for you, but it fills you up more quickly, which helps prevent you from overeating and consuming too many calories.

18. Life-Extending Anti-Aging Herbs

Herbs have been used for over 4,000 years to treat a wide variety of illnesses and ailments. Herbs are plants (NOT drugs) that contain potent antioxidants, vitamins, minerals, and enzymes. Used for their culinary, cosmetic, medicinal, and anti-aging purposes—herbs are shown to alleviate a host of age related conditions to maintain health, beauty, and longevity.

12 of the Most Popular Anti-Aging Herbs:

Ashwagandha - Traditionally used in Indian Ayurvedic medicine** for its rejuvenation and longevity enhancers—Ashwagandha promotes physical and mental health, reducing inflammation, stress, and high cholesterol. It's also known to improve immune system and sexual enhancement.

Chinese Wolfberry (Goji Berries) - Considered to be the world's most nutritious fruit—goji berries are extremely high in antioxidants, and have 500 times more vitamin-C per ounce than orange juice. These berries enhance vision health, stimulate the immune system, and protect the liver.

Ginkgo Biloba - High in antioxidants—ginkgo biloba is shown to alleviate age related memory loss. Used commonly for treatment in early-stage Alzheimer's disease,

93

this powerful herb enhances blood flow, not only to the brain, but throughout the entire body. Ginkgo's other anti-aging benefits include reducing stress, anxiety, and restoring energy.

Ginseng - One of the most widely used herbal supplements—ginseng is a well-know energy tonic (but without the jitters), which reduces fatigue and both emotional and physical stress. This energy booster enhances memory and strengthens the immune system. Ginseng is also found in many natural herbal anti-aging skin care products.

Gotu Kola - Used for centuries as a healing treatment—gotu kola is a nerve tonic which promotes relaxation and enhances memory. Sometimes confused with kola nut, gotu kola is non-stimulating and contains no caffeine. It's known for enhancing blood flow, especially to the legs, which helps in the prevention of varicose veins. It also helps the health of skin, hair, and nails and aids in many types of wound healing, as well as skin conditions such as eczema and psoriasis.

Grape Seed Extract - One of the most powerful antioxidants—this anti-aging herb promotes brain, skin, and eye health. It also helps improve cardiovascular health, improves mental health, and prevents senility. Grape seed extract is also used in cancer prevention.

Jiaolgulan (jow-goo-lawn) - Known as the "Immortality Herb," jiaolgulan is one of the major adaptogens** (a plant derivative). Jiaolgulan supports circulation and the immune system, lowers cholesterol and high blood pressure, modulates the nervous system, increases cardiac function, and normalizes cardiovascular and hormonal systems.

Maca - This powerful antioxidant and anti-carcinogen has a number of anti-aging benefits. Maca helps to regulate and maintain endocrine health. In addition, it enhances fertility, improves sexual function in both men and women, reduces hormonal dysfunction, and has been shown to enhance energy, endurance, and stamina.

Red Clover - Considered to be one of the richest sources of isoflavones (chemicals that act like estrogen), red clover is used for menopausal symptoms such as hot flashes and night sweats. It improves blood circulation, lowers cholesterol, and helps to prevent osteoporosis. This anti-aging herb also aids in digestion, helps with respiratory ailments, and improves liver health.

Reishi Mushroom - This mood elevating herbal supplement has anti-inflammatory, anti-viral, anti-allergic, and antioxidant properties. In addition, reishi mushrooms lower blood pressure, strengthens the immune system, and improves liver function.

Rhodiola Rosea - This anti-aging adaptogen enhances mental and physical performance, while improving cognitive function and fatigue. Rhodiola is well known for its anti-stress related capabilities. Many people are not aware that high stress living can cause chronic disease and premature aging. Rhodiola is one of the best herbs you can take if you lead a high stress lifestyle.

Schizandra - Known by Chinese women as a sexual enhancer (for both men and women) and youth tonic, schizandra improves adrenal health and lung, liver, and kidney function. This herb is mildly calming and has pain alleviating properties. It also purifies the blood, sharpens the mind, and improves memory.

NOTE: When first using herbs, some people may experience some cleansing action of the body (such as nausea, diarrhea, headaches, etc.). This is a temporary detoxing process that takes place while the body is being restored to health. If you have any health issues or concerns, it's best to check with your doctor, or holistic practitioner before starting any kind of home treatment.

**Adaptogens - Natural plant products that increase energy and endurance, reduces stress levels, promotes greater mental alertness, and has a balancing effect on body functions.

**Ayervedic Medicine - Ayervedic is a natural system of healing that originated in India more than 5,000 years ago. This holistic approach to healing is designed to improve and maintain health through diet, detoxification, yoga, breathing exercises, massage therapy, meditation, and herbal remedies by balancing mind, body, and spirit.

19. Improve Brain Health & Performance

The human brain contains roughly 80 to 120 billion brain cells (neurons). Poor diet, chronic tress, smoking, excessive alcohol use, and certain drugs can accelerate brain cell death.

The brain, much like a muscle, needs to work out to stay healthy and fit. The brain is hard at work 24 hours a day, every day. It determines how we think, how we feel, and how we act, as well as our emotional well-being. The brain is responsible for monitoring and regulating involuntary and voluntary actions in the body and is the intellectual center that allows thought, learning, memory, and creativity.

As we age, we begin to lose some of our brain power. Brain function and processing speed begins to slow down typically around age 40, but as early as age 30. It's estimated that over 60% of people eventually experience some loss of mental lucidity, as well as cognitive function, including memory loss, lack of concentration, thought clarity, focus, and judgement.

The Good News is... By challenging and pushing your brain, the stronger and healthier it becomes. Evidence shows, there are steps we can take to keep our brain sharp, healthy, and young, while reducing our risk for Alzheimer's disease or dementia.

Ways to Restore Brain Health:

Stay Mentally Active - To stay mentally sharp, it's important to work your mental muscles each and every day. To increase brain function, get involved in something that keeps your brain active. Take up a musical instrument, an art class, learn a new language, or challenge your brain with crossword or sudoku puzzles. Any activity that involves concentration will help exercise the mind and keep it young and sharp. Also, switch hands for 5 minutes a day. If you're right handed, use your left and vice versa. This simple exercise has been shown to develop the opposite side of your brain.

Stop Multi-Tasking - Taking the time to really pay close attention and focusing on just one task at a time, helps the brain store the information better, and recall it more easily at a later date.

Stay Physically Active - Exercise is not only good for the body, but it is good for the brain. Regular exercise improves memory, enhances cognitive function, clears brain fog, and slows down the loss of gray matter (the part of the brain that atrophies as we age).

Opt for a Brain Healthy Diet - Consuming a diet low in saturated fats and cholesterol and rich in healthy fats like omega-3 fatty acids, complex carbohydrates, lean protein, and high in antioxidants—protects brain cells and are essential to brain function.

Brain Healthy Supplements - Omega-3 fatty acids found in cold water fish like salmon or tuna, or taken in supplement form are considered by many experts to be the most important ingredient for optimal brain health.

Researchers have found that fish oil contains many essential nutrients that help brain function. Gingko biloba is also one of the most commonly used supplements for brain health, as it increases blood flow to the brain.

Avoid Substances that Stress the Brain - Caffeine, cigarette smoking, excessive alcohol consumption, refined sugars, and recreational drugs all decrease blood flow to the brain, which can increase your risk of dementia and cognitive decline and can cause premature aging.

Get Enough Sleep - Getting a good nights sleep is crucial for proper brain function. Studies show that people who are sleep-deprived and don't get enough sleep, have more trouble absorbing and retaining new information than those who are well rested. **NOTE:** For more information on how to get a good nights sleep—please refer to tip # 9.

100

20. Break Unhealthy Bad Habits

While we may not want to admit it, most of us have at least one bad habit (or two). And while some bad habits, such as knuckle cracking, skin picking, or nail biting are just downright irksome for ourselves, as well as other people—bad habits such as excessive drinking or smoking can pose serious health risks.

If you're serious about your long term health and anti-aging, as well as your looks—cutting back on alcohol consumption and/or quitting smoking are at the top of the list of the most monumental health decisions you can make.

Harmful Effects on the Body - While many people think cigarette smoking helps them relax and cope with the stresses of daily life, the truth is, smoking does just the opposite. With each puff of the cigarette, you're putting your body into a state of physical stress—sending over four thousand poisonous gasses, toxic metals, and carci-nogenic chemicals racing through your bloodstream, affecting everything from your blood pressure, to the health of your organs.

In addition to the major health concerns such as lung cancer, heart disease, and emphysema—smoking is associated with higher levels of chronic inflammation, as well as an increase in free radicals, which weakens the immune system, while depleting the body of protective antioxidants.

For Skin Health - Smoking is second to overexposure to the sun for making skin look old, sallow, wrinkled, leathery, and unhealthy—a condition known as smoker's face. Smoking depletes the collagen in the skin, causing significantly more wrinkling and less elasticity to the skin than non-smokers, while discoloring the teeth, which is often associated with aging.

Common Sense Recommendation - If you're serious about getting your health on track, looking younger, and feeling your best, while adding quality years to your life... you owe it to yourself to quit smoking!

21. Prevent Osteoporosis Through Diet & Lifestyle

Osteoporosis is often referred to as the "silent disease" because it has no symptoms. Osteoporosis (which means porous bone) is a condition which causes bone to become weak and brittle.

Bone health is determined by diet, exercise, dietary supplements, as well as lifestyle. It's estimated that roughly 10 million people in the United States alone have osteoporosis, and 80% of them are women. Another 30+ million have low bone density, putting them at a greater risk of developing osteoporosis. In addition... more than 1.5 million people suffer broken bones (mainly hip and spine fractures) each year due to osteoporosis and brittle bones.

NOT Just an Elderly Disease - Doctors report that they're seeing an increase in signs of osteoporosis in women as young as 20 years of age. They believe the spike in younger women, is because of poor dietary habits that develop during childhood. More kids are now drinking soda pop, instead of milk, and are not getting the calcium and vitamin-D, as well as other nutrients needed during their prime bone-building years.

Steps You Can Take to Combat Osteoporosis:

Women are more apt to develop osteoporosis than men, because the drop in estrogen levels during menopause exacerbates bone loss. After menopause, women lose about 1-2% of their bone density each year.

Also, if you're lacking certain bone building vitamins and minerals, this can also play a significant role in the onset of osteoporosis. By adopting and maintaining a healthy lifestyle, and making sure you get adequate levels of calcium and magnesium, you can keep osteoporosis at bay, while keeping your bones strong and healthy.

Consuming a calcium-rich diet is an ideal way to build and maintain strong bones. Physical activity is another key preventive measure. Using your muscles actually helps protect your bones. Low impact aerobic exercise like brisk walking, climbing stairs, hiking, swimming, dancing, playing tennis, and bike riding—along with strength training exercise using light weights, has been shown to strengthen bones, while increasing bone density.

You're at Risk of Osteoporosis if...

- You're a female between the age of 20-100

- Osteoporosis runs in your family

- You're post-menopausal

- You've had a hysterectomy or chemotherapy

- You are thin and petite

- You have, or have had an eating disorder such as Anorexia or Bulimia

- You consume a diet low in calcium & vitamin-D

- You smoke

- You drink alcohol or caffeine in excess

- You don't exercise

- You have mercury poisoning (toxicity)

- You are Caucasian or Asian (Black and Hispanic women have a lower risk)

Bone Building Vitamins - Premenopausal women should consume 1,000 milligrams of calcium a day preferably through diet and/or in supplement form, plus 400-800 IU of vitamin-D, which helps the body to absorb calcium. Postmenopausal women require even more— 1,200-1,500 milligrams of calcium and 800-1,000 IU of vitamin-D per day. In addition, it's important to also add 300-500 milligrams of chelated magnesium daily. The best supplements contain both calcium and magnesium together.

NOTE: If you think you may be at risk for developing osteoporosis, schedule a Bone Mineral Density (BMD) test with your doctor. If you are overweight, by losing just 10-20 lbs. you can substantially reduce your risk of developing osteoporosis.

22. Arthritis Prevention: Life Without Pain

The word arthritis means "joint inflammation" or "damage to the joints," which result in pain, swelling, stiffness, and limited movement. Some varieties of arthritis can extend to the muscles, organs, as well as the skin. It's most common in adults 65 and older, but can affect people of all ages, including children.

There are over 100 types of arthritis that collectively affect over 45 million adults in the United States alone, but the two most common are osteoarthritis and rheumatoid. Arthritis involves the breakdown of cartilage which protects the joints. Arthritis frequently occurs in the hands and fingers, feet, knees, spine, and hips. Some of the factors that may cause arthritis are genetics, age, excessive body weight, previous injury, broken bones, autoimmune disease, trauma from an accident, and general wear and tear on the joints.

Natural Treatments for Arthritis - Treatments range from acupuncture, magnetic therapy, heat and/or cold compresses, body massage, steam baths, relaxation remedies, and stress reducing activities such as mediation, yoga, qigong, or tai chi. Infrared saunas have a passive cardiovascular conditioning effect and have been shown to benefit people who suffer from arthritis pain. More and more studies show that regular exercise and other kinds of activities can help people who suffer from arthritis.

In Addition... There are many alternatives to prescription drugs, such as taking natural supplements like glucosamine, chondroitin, as well as anti-inflammatory herbal extracts like turmeric and ginger. Studies also show that taking omega-3 fatty acids (fish oil) can significantly improve pain, stiffness, and swelling of arthritic joints.

Part III:

6 Anti-Aging Foods That Offer a Powerhouse of Nutrition

For centuries now, man has been on the lookout for tonics and potions that can slow down the aging process. There are so many little things we can do to turn back the clock and to delay, or prevent age-related conditions and/or illnesses, including eating certain foods that boost immunity and fight disease.

Eating nutrient dense foods enables you to fulfill your requirements for essential fatty acids, essential amino acids, proteins, vitamins, minerals, and antioxidants. These nutritional powerhouses are not processed and do not contain synthetic or artificial ingredients.

Add These 6 Natural, Power-Packed Super Food Sources Into Your Daily Diet for Added Nutrition, Health, and Longevity Benefits:

23. Hemp, Chia & Flax: Seeds of Life

(a) Hemp Seed

Hemp originated in Central Asia over 12,000 years ago and was grown for its fiber, oil, and seeds. Not to be confused with marijuana—hemp is in the marijuana family, but contains only microscopic levels of THC, and WILL NOT get you high. Instead, hemp seed is considered to be one of the world's most nutritious seeds, and one of the most easily digested foods on earth.

Hemp seeds are not only delicious, but are a superior source of protein, as well as a rich source of essential fatty acids and essential amino acids. Hemp seed also comes in oil form and can be used on salads, in smoothies, etc., as well as topically on the skin. Hemp seed oil is non-greasy, very healing, and an excellent anti-aging moisturizer.

Hemp Seeds Many Health and Healing Benefits:

- Supports a Healthy Metabolism

- Facilitates Fat Burning

- Helps Lower Bad LDL & High Cholesterol

- Reduces Hormonal Symptoms

- Decreases Inflammatory Conditions

- Regulates the Digestive System

- Supports Healthy Hair, Nail, and Skin Health

- Reduces Food Cravings & Promotes Weight Loss

NOTE: Hemp seed is found to be completely safe for those who have allergies or an intolerance to gluten or nuts.

(b) Chia Seed

Chia is a member of the mint family, grown for its seed in Southern Mexico and Guatemala. Chia has been used for its medicinal and healing properties as early as 3500 BC. These nutty tasting whole grain chia seeds are one of the healthiest anti-aging superfoods available and are considered to be one of nature's perfect foods. The chia seed is an excellent source of fiber, antioxidants, protein, vitamins, minerals, and is one of the highest sources of omega-3 fatty acids on the planet. This powerful gluten-free seed is extremely versatile—it can be eaten raw, cooked, sprouted, ground, or as a gel.

Chia Seeds Many Health and Healing Benefits:

- Promotes Cardiovascular Health

- Promotes Bone Health

- Stabilizes Blood Sugar

- Boosts Brain Function

- Improves Digestive Health

- Improves Mental Focus & Concentration

- Regulates Blood Pressure

- Increases Endurance and Energy Levels

- Reduces Menopausal Symptoms

- Gluten Free

- Promotes Healthy Elimination & Detoxification

Chia for Weight Loss - Beside their nutritional value, chia seeds are also an effective aid for healthy weight loss. When the chia seed is exposed to water, it has the ability to absorb more than twelve times its weight in water. This produces a gelatinous substance, which when ingested, creates a feeling of fullness. This helps suppress the appetite and eliminate food cravings. The chia seed is also known to reduce cravings for sweets and junk food, while promoting lean muscle mass.

(c) Flax Seed

Originating in Mesopotamia (modern day southern Iraq) —flax seeds health, healing, and medicinal purposes have been known for thousands of years. Flax seed comes in 2 basic varieties—brown and yellow (or golden). While brown and golden flax seed have similar nutritional value, golden is touted as having a superior flavor.

Flax seed (or flaxseed) is high in fiber (both soluble and insoluble), protein, vitamins and minerals, as well as a balanced ratio of omega-3, 6, and 9 fatty acids. It also contains high levels of natural antioxidants, known as lignans. Lignans are plant-based substances (phytochemicals) that act like human estrogen. Lignans are found in the fiber portion of flax seed and have remarkable health benefits. Flax seed contains up to 800 times more lignans than any other plant food.

Flax Seeds Many Health and Healing Benefits:

- Promotes Cardiovascular Health

- Boosts Immune System

- Lowers Cholesterol

- Stabilizes Blood Sugar Levels

- Helps Prevent Breast, Colon, & Prostate Cancer

- Aids in Digestion

- Helps Prevent Inflammatory Bowel Syndrome

- Helps Prevent Crohn's Disease

- Helps Prevent Colitis

- Protects Against Type 2 Diabetes

- Reduces Arthritis Inflammation

- Helps Prevent Macular Degeneration

- Reduces Menopausal Symptoms

- Alleviates Symptoms of Psoriasis

Flax for Weight Loss - Flax increases the body's metabolic rate, which helps to burn fat, and it's high fiber content helps fill you up, so you consume fewer calories.

Whole vs. Ground - Flax seed is available as whole seeds, ground seeds, and oil. To achieve the most benefits from flax seed, nutritionists recommend consuming ground flax seed over whole, as whole flax seeds do not digest well. **NOTE:** If you do purchase whole flax seed, grind it up first in a food processor or coffee grinder.

How Much Flax Do You Need? Just 2 tablespoons a day of ground flax seed is all you need for it's amazing health and nutritional benefits. Flax seed has a delicious nutty flavor and can be consumed in fruit smoothies, or sprinkled on cereal, oatmeal, yogurt, or salad.

24. Extra-Virgin Olive Oil: A Powerful Age Reversing Elixir

A key ingredient in the Mediterranean diet—extra virgin olive oils many health and longevity benefits date back to over 5,000 years ago. In the Mediterranean countries (Greece, Italy, and Spain) where extra-virgin olive oil is not only a staple, but the main fat used, rates of chronic diseases are lower than in any other cultures.

All Olive Oils Are Not Created Equal - Extra-virgin olive oil (sometimes referred to as EVOO) is considered to be one of the world's healthiest foods. Extra-virgin olive oil is a rich source of heart-healthy mono-unsaturated fats and contains the highest levels of antioxidants in comparison to virgin or pure olive oils.

The 4 Main Types of Olive Oils:

Pure Olive Oil - The name can be misleading, as pure olive oil is actually a refined olive oil blended with a touch of virgin or extra-virgin olive oil for flavor. Chemically refined and filtered—pure olive oil is the least expensive and lowest quality. **NOTE:** The refining process removes much of the flavor, aroma, and natural antioxidants.

Light Olive Oil - Light olive oil is essentially the same thing as pure olive oil. **NOTE:** The term "light" refers to it's color, flavor, and aroma—not to it's caloric content.

Virgin Olive Oil - Virgin is the olive oil produced from the second pressing. Produced without any chemical additives—virgin olive oil contains no refined oil and has an acidity (fatty acids) level of less that 2%.

Extra-Virgin Olive Oil - Extra-virgin olive oil is the purest form of olive oil—extracted from the olive fruit using only gentle pressure and warm water, through a process known as cold pressing. There is no heat or chemicals used in the extraction process. EVOO is the oil that comes from the first pressing of the olives and has an acidity level of 0.8% or lower. To be considered extra virgin, the acidity level must not exceed 0.8%. EVOO is the highest quality oil, with a superior blend of flavor and aroma.

Extra-Virgin Olive Oil Provides Numerous Health, Healing, and Anti-Aging Benefits:

- Reduces the Risk of Heart Disease

- Promotes Healthy Digestion

- Cancer Prevention (Breast, Colon, and Prostate)

- Lowers Risk of Stroke

- Lowers Risk of Type 2 Diabetes

- Lowers Blood Pressure

- Lowers Bad Cholesterol (LDL)

- Raises Good Cholesterol (HDL)

- Improves Cognitive Function

- Improves Bone Health**

A Natural Inflammatory - Because EVOO is a natural inflammatory, it also benefits those suffering from osteoporosis, rheumatoid arthritis, and asthma. **EVOO is highly recommended for the elderly, as it stimulates bone mineralization, preventing calcium loss.

EVOO for Obesity - Although high in calories, extra-virgin olive oil has been shown to reduce levels of obesity and slow down age-related weight gain. EVOO also acts as an appetite suppressant, which leads to fewer calories consumed at mealtime.

EVOO for Depression - Research shows that a diet rich in extra-virgin olive oil can have a significant impact on our mental health and for those suffering from depression. **NOTE:** Reduce your intake of foods containing trans and saturated fats (found in fast and processed foods) to lower your risk of developing depression.

Americans Need an Oil Change - Substitute extra-virgin olive oil in place of saturated fats and refined vegetable oils for a much healthier alternative. Just 1-2 tablespoons of EVOO a day is all you need to bolster your immune system and reap it's many health, healing, and longevity benefits.

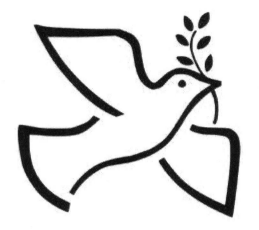

25. Acai Berry: Nature's Energy Fruit

Harvested in the rainforest of South America, acai is considered to be one of the most nutritious foods there is. Acai (pronounced: ah-sy-EE) is a high-energy berry that tastes like a blend of berries and chocolate. Acai contains an extremely high concentration of amino acids, antioxidants, and omega-3, 6, and 9 essential fatty acids that help combat premature aging and provides the body with excellent anti-bacterial and anti-viral protection.

 # 1 Superfood - Research shows that the acai berry has more antioxidant power than blueberries, cranberries, blackberries, raspberries, or strawberries. In fact, this little purple berry is said to contain the highest levels of antioxidants of any fruit or berry in the world to date, and has been called the number one superfood for optimal health. There are a number of reasons to add acai supplements or acai juice to your daily diet plan.

The Many Health and Healing Benefits of Acai:

- Boosts the Immune System

- Increases Energy and Stamina

- Improves Cardiovascular Health

- Acts as a Powerful Anti-Inflammatory

- Helps Combat Illness and Disease

- Detoxifies the Body

- Promotes Healthy Skin and Hair

- Promotes Brain Health

- Elevates Mood

- Reduces Cholesterol

- Improves Sexual Function

- Promotes Weight Loss

Acai for Healthy Skin and Hair - In recent years, because of it's powerful healing and rejuvenating properties, acai has become increasingly popular as an age defying ingredient found in many skin care, hair care, and cosmetic products. So, whether you use acai internally, externally, or both—discover the amazing, beautifying, and healthful benefits of the acai berry.

26. Aloe Vera: The Multi-Purpose Miracle Plant

This powerful natural healer has been used for over 4,000 years for its medicinal benefits, as well as its soothing and anti-inflammatory properties. The aloe vera plant is about 95% water—the rest of the plant contains potent levels of essential oils, essential fatty acids, amino acids, enzymes, vitamins, and minerals.

Aloe vera gel is ideal for topical use on burns, wounds, abrasions, as well as chronic skin conditions like eczema and psoriasis. For internal use, aloe vera has natural detoxifying properties that work to cleanse and heal the digestive system. Topically, aloe vera is one of the most popular and effective ingredients found in skin care products and cosmetics.

Additional Health and Healing Benefits of Aloe Vera:

- Alleviates Inflammation

- Boosts the Immune System

- Relieves Constipation

- Relieves Acid Reflux and Heartburn

- Increases Energy and Stamina

- Detoxifies the Liver, Kidneys, Colon and Blood

- Treats Gum Disease

- Contains Antibacterial & Antifungal Properties

- Contains Antiseptic Properties

- Acts as a Pain Inhibitor

- Effective Treatment for Peptic Ulcers

- Treats Irritable Bowel Syndrome (IBS)

- Promotes Healthy Weight Loss

- Rebuilds Collagen and Elastin

- Extremely Moisturizing to the Skin

- Effective in Reducing Wrinkles & Stretch Marks

- Effective in Reducing Hyperpigmentation

- Reduces the Signs of Aging

Flavorless vs. Bitter - Whether you use aloe vera internally, or for external use—aloe vera is considered to be one of the most versatile and effective natural healers. When using it as an internal dietary supplement, drink 2 oz. of aloe vera juice twice daily. Aloe vera juice can be taken alone or mixed with juice. Up until recently, most aloe vera juices had a bitter taste, which may be considered somewhat unpleasant. Nowadays, you can find flavorless aloe vera juice, which tastes just like pure spring water.

27. Apple Cider Vinegar: Harness it's Healing Powers

Raw organic apple cider vinegar is a powerful health tonic that has been used throughout history for its anti-septic, antifungal, and antibacterial healing and natural medicinal benefits. It's been recorded that Hippocrates (The Father of Medicine) used apple cider vinegar as far back as 400 BC for its many cleansing and healing components. Rich in anti-aging antioxidants, vitamins, minerals, potassium, calcium, pectin, malic acid, and antioxidants—apple cider vinegar is extremely effective in detoxifying the body, while purifying both the blood stream and vital organs. Apple cider vinegar is also a highly effective home remedy for a number of ailments.

Apple Cider Vinegar is Used to Treat a Variety of Health Issues Both Internally and Externally:

- Strengthens the Immune System

- Increases Energy and Stamina

- Lowers High Blood Pressure and Cholesterol

- Reduces Chronic Fatigue

- Promotes Digestion and pH balance

- Reduces Heartburn and Indigestion

- Helps Detoxify the Body

- Helps with Constipation

- Fights Allergies in Humans and Pets

- Reduces Sinus Infections

- Cures Yeast Infections

- Alleviates Symptoms of Arthritis and Gout

- Helps Treat Skin Conditions Like Acne & Eczema

Organic, Raw, and Unfiltered is the One to Buy - The best type of apple cider vinegar to use is "mother of vinegar," which can be found in health food stores and is made from unpasteurized, organically grown apples.

Relief from Varicose Veins - Apple cider vinegar is said to reduce the appearance of varicose veins. The treatment requires applying a cloth soaked with full strength apple cider vinegar to the affected areas twice a day for 30 minutes, while lying down with your feet elevated.

Weight Loss Benefits - Apple cider vinegar is also known to break down fat in the body and is widely used for weight loss. Just mix 2 tsps. of apple cider vinegar with an 8 oz. glass of water and drink before meals or sip throughout the day. This healthy weight-loss concoction helps suppress appetite while revving up the metabolism.

An Apple a Day Keeps the Doctor Away - Consume this "apple cider vinegar elixir" to boost your immune system and for overall health. Mix 1 tablespoon apple cider vinegar, 2 tsp. raw honey, a squeeze of fresh lemon juice, and a dash of cinnamon mixed in an 8 oz. glass of water for an energizing tonic and powerful healing elixir.

28. Green Tea: The Natural Healing Brew

Discovered in China over 4,000 years ago, the Chinese have been enjoying this brew ever since for its anti-aging, health, beauty, and medicinal purposes. Green tea is used to treat digestive problems, depression, enhance energy, boost the immune system, and to prolong life. Unlike black tea, green tea is not fermented, instead the active components remain in the herb. Green tea contains a variety of chemical compounds, minerals, vitamins, and is rich in anti-aging antioxidants.

Green Tea's Many Health Benefits - There are a number of health and anti-aging benefits which can result from the regular consumption. Green tea protects against cardiovascular disease, all forms of cancer, free radical damage and cellular damage, while reducing bad cholesterol, high blood pressure, blood sugar levels, and risk of stroke. Green tea has been shown to prevent the death of brain cells, which means less chance of dementia, Alzheimer's, or Parkinson's disease.

Green Tea for Natural Weight Loss - Green tea is also excellent for promoting the growth of friendly bacteria in the intestines, while encouraging loss of abdominal fat, and increasing greater physical stamina. Green tea's powerful antioxidants help rev up the metabolism, while effectively boosting calorie and fat burning.

How Much Green Tea Should You Drink? 2-4 cups of caffeine-free green tea a day is recommended for it's many amazing health benefits, as well as for disease prevention. If you drink the caffeinated version and consume more than the recommended amount, it may cause heart palpitations. For added health benefits and a little sweetness, add a teaspoon of manuka honey

Regular Honey vs. Manuka Honey - Manuka honey is a very special and rare type of honey that contains significantly higher levels of vitamins, minerals, antioxidants, and amino acids than any other type of honey. Manuka honey, which is often regarded as a medicinal food, comes from the nectar of the manuka plant grown in New Zealand, and is only harvested for 6 weeks out of the entire year. This raw organic honey can be used both internally and externally for its many healing benefits and contains natural antiseptic, antibacterial, antiviral, antifungal, and anti-inflammatory components.

Treat Yourself to a Tea Bath - For a wonderful home-spa treatment that you can experience at any time, pamper yourself by taking a relaxing herbal green tea bath! Just fill the tub with tepid water and throw in 3-4 bags of green tea and a few drops of chamomile or lavender essential oils. The tannins and powerful antioxidants are extremely beneficial and anti-aging to the skin.

Part IV:

5 Anti-Aging Tips That Work Like Magic

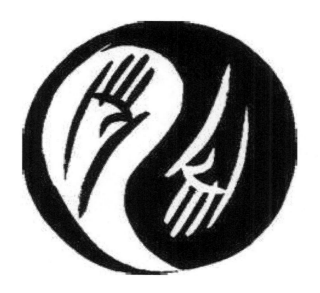

Many baby boomers are electing to go under the knife in their quest to look younger and improve their appearance. While it's true that cosmetic surgery can do wonders for your looks—cosmetic surgery is costly, painful, and does not come without risks.

Fortunately, there are a number of ways to naturally enhance and transform your appearance without cosmetic
surgery, and without spending a fortune?

These natural anti-aging tips will brighten your eyes, lift
those sagging jowls and droopy eyelids, eliminate
wrinkles, reduce stress, enhance your self-esteem, and
have you looking younger, fresher, and feeling absolutely
fabulous in no time!

**Improve Your Natural Beauty and Boost Your Self-
Confidence, Without Cosmetic Surgery, With These
Anti-Aging, Health, & Beauty Tips:**

29. Facial Exercise: The Natural Facelift

Do you look older than you feel? Wrinkles, loose skin on the neck (turkey neck), and sagging jowls are some of the most hated effects of aging. They can give the appearance of being old and tired, and can greatly impact the way we feel about ourselves. Fortunately, there is a solution. Facial exercise is a natural cost-effective way to achieve a non-surgical face lift, without the pain of surgery, and without breaking the bank.

Face Lift Through Exercise - Facial exercise benefits the entire face, as well as the neck. It reduces fine lines and wrinkles, lifts sagging jowls, minimizes puffy eyes and dark circles, reduces a double chin, lifts droopy eyelids, and eliminates crow's feet. In addition, it increases collagen and elastin production, stimulates blood circulation, oxygenates the skin cells, and hydrates the skin.

Detoxify Your Skin - Another important benefit of facial exercise is the draining of excess lymph. At night time, while we're sleeping, toxins can form and waste builds up. Facial exercise can help facilitate lymph drainage, while helping improve blood circulation, which has a detoxifying effect on facial skin. This improves the appearance of the complexion by clearing impurities and dead skin cells, while reducing excess fluids and overall puffiness, particularly around the most obvious area, the eyes.

Causes of Puffy Eyes - Puffy eyes can be caused by a number of factors including: fluid retention, excess salt in your diet, allergies, stress, hormonal fluctuations, too little sleep, excessive alcohol intake, and not drinking enough water. **NOTE:** For more information on alleviating puffy eyes and dark circles—please refer to tip # 30.

Bottom Line: By following a good skin care regimen and performing a facial exercise regimen just a few days a week, you'll be amazed just how much younger and more refreshed you'll look.

30. Hydrotherapy: For Healthy, Youthful, Vibrant Eyes

Look in the mirror at your eyes. Are they bright and clear, or do they look old and tired? If you suffer from eye fatigue, tired eyes, or computer vision syndrome (CVS), hydrotherapy (aka water therapy) is a natural and very soothing method of healing eye discomfort, while helping to restore eye health.

Hydrotherapy will rejuvenate and nourish your eyes, making the white's whiter, your eyes brighter, clearer, and totally refreshed.

Alternate Back and Forth - Hydrotherapy treatments are performed by holding hot and cold water compresses against the eyes for 30-60 seconds each, repeating 3-4 times. The hot application expands the blood vessels in the eyes, while the cold restricts the blood vessels. Start with the hot compress and end with the cold. After your hydrotherapy session, your eyes will look and feel like new! **NOTE:** Make sure the compress is not too hot, as to burn your skin!

For Dark Circles and Puffy Under Eye Bags - Green, black, or chamomile tea is a natural solution for helping minimize dark circles and puffy eyes. These teas contain tannins, a natural astringent that constricts blood vessels, reduces inflammation, and swelling. Prepare two bags of tea by steeping them in boiling water, wringing them out, and chilling them in the refrigerator or freezer. Place the chilled tea bag over your (closed) eyes for 10-15 minutes, turning them over half way through.

For Good Eye Health - Proper nutrition is vital for keeping your eyes healthy and functioning at optimal level. Two important nutrients (carotenoids) that may help lower the risk of vision impairments and age-related chronic eye conditions like cataracts and macular degeneration are leutine (LOO teen) and zeaxanthin (zee ah ZAN thin).

Nutrition For the Eyes - For healthy eyes, eat foods rich in omega-3 fatty acids along with foods high in antioxidants like vitamins A, C, and E and minerals, zinc and selenium. Consume plenty of deep colored fruit and vegetables, which are a good source of beta-carotene and contain an abundance of carotenoids. Green and yellow vegetables such as broccoli, spinach, bell peppers, turnip greens, kale, carrots, sweet potatoes, and pumpkin—and fruits like oranges, grapefruit, lemons, kiwi, strawberries, blueberries, apricots, and mangoes.

Other Good Forms of Ocular Nutrition Include... Spices like garlic, basil, oregano, paprika, turmeric, and parsley and herbs such as bilberry, passionflower, gingko biloba, and golden seal.

31. DIY Scalp Massage: Relax & Stimulate

A good head and scalp massage not only feels incredible, but has many health and healing benefits for your entire body. When the scalp is massaged, the rest of the body relaxes, too. Massaging the scalp stimulates the nerves and blood vessels, sending tingling sensations from the scalp to the toes. It relieves tension, provides deep relaxation, lubricates and conditions the scalp, strengthens and nourishes the hair root to stimulate hair growth, and helps prevent hair loss.

A soothing head and scalp massage provides instant relief from stress, depression, headaches, and pain. And don't think you have to go to a salon or spa to get a scalp massage—you can perform one on yourself using warmed aromatherapy essential oils like peppermint, rosemary, lavender, or virgin coconut. **NOTE:** For more information on essential and carrier oils—please refer to tip # 47.

Melt Away Stress Using Your Own Finger Tips - Using a few drops of essential oils on your finger tips, start by running your fingers through your hair using slight pressure, from the front to the back of the head. Then perform with circular motions—repeating the process starting at the base of the skull, moving up to the top of the head. Next, start from the sides—massage from the temples and ears all the way up to the top of the head, then to the front of the head, and then back to the base of the skull. Repeat with gentle circular motions. Finish up with gentle hair tugging. Simply slip your fingers through your hair and gently tug at the roots, holding for a few seconds and then letting go.

NOTE: Depending on your preference, a scalp massage can be performed on wet or dry hair, and can be performed with or without the use of essential oils.

Minimize Hair Loss - Maximize Regrowth - Daily scalp massage is not only beneficial for stress and relaxation, but helps stimulate new hair growth, while stopping thinning hair, and reversing hair loss. **NOTE:** For more information on thinning hair and hair loss—please refer to tip # 33.

32. Skin Needling: Anti-Aging Skin Rejuvenation Treatment

Skin needling, also known as micro-needling, is the newest, easiest, and one of the most effective anti-aging skin care rejuvenation treatments available today! Performed in clinics or as an at-home treatment, skin needling delivers equivalent results to laser resurfacing, chemical peels, and dermabrasion treatments, but at a fraction of the cost! This non-invasive treatment is a form of Collagen Induction Therapy (CIT), improving the skin's health and beauty by stimulating and replenishing collagen production in record time, and without damage to the skin.

Skin Needling Can be Performed on the Face, Neck, Body and Scalp and Has Been Shown to:

- Reduce and Smooth Fine Lines & Wrinkles

- Repair Sun Damaged Skin & Skin Discolorations

- Thicken and Repair Thin Crepey Skin

- Increase the Effectiveness of Skin Care Products

- Visibly Reduce Acne and Surgical Scarring

- Tighten and Lift Sagging Skin

- Help Lift and Elevate the Eye Brows

- Reduce Pore Size

- Improve Skin Texture

- Improve the Appearance of Stretch Marks

- Improve the Appearance of Cellulite

- Reduce and Restore Hair Loss & Hair Thinning

How Does Skin Needling Work? Skin needling is implemented through the use of a skin roller. The skin roller is a hand-held device containing very tiny, fine needles. As the device is rolled over the skin, this causes microscopic puncture wounds that penetrate the outer layer of skin into the dermis. This causes very minute injury to the skin and immediately signals the body's own healing mechanisms to stimulate new collagen and elastin production. The results imitate those obtained with a laser, but without causing trauma to the epidermis. The healing period is very rapid, and the holes usually close within one hour, but the production of collagen continues up to 12 months after the procedure.

Is Skin Needling Painful? - If you're using a home-use skin roller it may be slightly uncomfortable at first, especially around sensitive areas like the nose, forehead, and upper lip, but your skin does quickly adapt. While tolerance levels do vary, by combining gentle pressure with the correct needle length, most people report feeling only tingling sensations and find it very tolerable.

NOTE: Medical skin needling for more severe conditions such as surgical scarring, deep pitted acne scars, chicken pox scars, and sun damage require a more aggressive approach, and a topical numbing cream is generally applied.

33. Stop Thinning Hair and Hair Loss

Not all women have long, thick, beautiful hair. As we age, thinning hair and hair loss are a very common complaint among older women. If you're shedding from 50 to 100 hairs a day, that is considered normal—but if you're seeing thinning on top of your head, bald spots, or experiencing thinning in your part line, it could be caused by a variety of factors. It's estimated that approximately 30 million women in America have thinning hair—that's roughly 1 in 4 women that suffer from female hair loss.

Common Causes for Women's Hair Loss Include:

Menopause - Whether you're menopausal or postmenopausal, losing hair is common due to hormonal changes and imbalances in the body, especially testosterone imbalances, which not only can lead to hair thinning and loss, but may also shrink hair follicles.

DHT - Dihydrotestosterone (DHT) is a hormonal by-product of testosterone, and is considered to be the main culprit for hair loss in both men and women. DHT is also responsible for shrinking and weakening the hair follicles, which result in the hair follicles growing smaller and deteriorating. **NOTE:** There are many DHT blockers for hair loss currently on the market which have shown promising results.

Stress - Emotional stress causes the adrenal glands to become overworked, and can lead to hormonal imbalances, which can wreak havoc on the body and can cause hair loss.

Highly Acidic Diet - Foods high in acid production like sugar, caffeine, animal proteins, and processed foods all throw off the body's pH balance, which can slow down hair growth and result in hair loss.

Medications - Certain medications used to treat depression, arthritis, high blood pressure, and heart problems, as well as birth control pills and diet pills containing amphetamines, can result in hair loss for some women.

Genetics - Known as female pattern baldness or alopecia—family history is a factor in hair loss. This type of hair loss can be devastating for women, as it tends to worsen as you age.

NOTE: Other causes of hair loss include: extreme dieting, lack of nutrition, certain medications and drugs, childbirth, and illnesses such as lupus, polycystic ovarian syndrome, and thyroid disease.

Hair Thinning and Hair Loss Remedies:

Volumizing Shampoo - Use a volumizing shampoo designed for thinning hair. Look for products that contain wheat protein to thicken hair.

DO NOT Use Maximum Hold Hairsprays -They tend to fracture the hair shaft as you brush it out. Opt for a flexible hold instead.

Say NO to Perms - Avoid permanent hair dyes, perming, bleaching, and chemical straightening solutions if you're prone to thinning hair and hair loss. Harsh products penetrate thinner hair more rapidly causing damage and breakage.

Avoid Putting Too Much Tension on the Hair - Too-tight pony tails and teasing all cause hair breakage. Over styling and excessive brushing can also damage the hair shaft and cause hair to fall out.

Diet - Your diet can play a major role in hair loss. Fad diets, crash diets, eating disorders, and certain illnesses can cause poor nutrition. Eating a wholesome, balanced diet with adequate protein and rich in silica, calcium, zinc, folic acid, amino acids, keratin, vitamins A, B, and C, and iron will help combat thinning hair and hair loss.

Scalp Massage - A scalp massage with aromatherapy essential oils is very effective for treating hair loss and hair thinning, as it stimulates the scalp and hair follicles, while promoting hair growth and a clean, healthy scalp.

Once a Week... Massage the entire scalp for four to five minutes using firm pressure. Use 2-3 drops of basil, clary sage, lavender, or rosemary essential oils combined with 1 teaspoon of a carrier oil such as jojoba, grapeseed, or hemp. These natural essential oils are all very effective for treating hair loss and thinning hair, as they simulate hair growth and thicken hair. Carrier oils are just as important as the essential oils—carrier oils provide essential fatty acids to the scalp and hair follicles. **NOTE:** For more information on scalp massage—please refer to tip # 31.

Skin Needling - When combined with a topical hair growth product, skin needling has shown excellent results for helping both men and women in stimulating hair growth and restoration. Skin needling can help with thinning hair, receding hairlines, bald spots, and alopecia. **NOTE:** For more information on skin needling—please refer to tip #32.

Laser Treatments - For those who prefer to opt for the latest in new technology, the Revage 670 Hair Restoration Laser boasts an 85% success rate. Revage is a cool laser that stops the progression of hair loss and promotes new hair growth in as little as 4-16 weeks. The laser treatments are performed 2-3 times a week for 20 minutes and are completely painless. The cost runs between $3,000 - $5,000 for 1 year of treatments, and then maintenance treatments are performed anywhere from once a month, up to once every three months.

NOTE: Many times female hair loss is temporary and may last only a few months. If you're experiencing unusually excessive hair loss, contact your doctor to discuss your symptoms and the appropriate treatment needed to restore hair growth.

Part V:

8 Anti-Aging Tips That Have a Profound Impact on Your Health

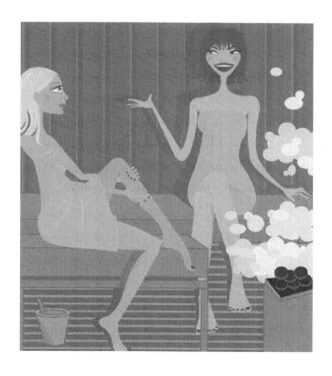

We expect certain changes to occur in our appearance and bodies as we grow older—graying hair, wrinkling of the skin, less energy, memory loss, decreased libido, etc. Not everyone welcomes these changes, at least without a fight. Wouldn't it be great if we could actually look more youthful and feel more energetic as we move into our golden years? Well, it is entirely possible! Aging can't be stopped, but by taking our health seriously and pursuing our health through positive lifestyle changes, we can discourage the aging process and add good quality years to our lives.

By incorporating the winning combination of these life changing and life enhancing tips and secrets, you'll find you have more energy, your skin will look fabulous, and you'll feel refreshed, energized, and rejuvenated!

Experience These Powerful Age-Defying Tips For Optimal Health and Boundless Energy:

34. Diaphragmatic: The Correct Way to Breathe

Breathing is the easiest exercise of all, yet a large majority of people do not know how to do it correctly. Instead, they are shallow "chest" breathers, using only a small portion of their lung capacity, when they should be breathing fully and deeply into their lower lungs. Shallow breathing robs the body of sufficient oxygen and is usually associated with stress, anxiety, panic disorders, high blood pressure, memory problems, sexual dysfunction, and depression.

Sit Up Straight - People with bad posture and who tend to slouch, generally are shallow breathers. Slouching compresses the diaphragm and organs, which limits the oxygen intake, causing stress to the body. Deep diaphragmatic breathing has a powerful impact on our health. By breathing deeply and fully, it revs up the heart rate, oxygenating every cell in the body, from the brain to all our vital organs.

The Power of Learning to Breathe Properly - Whether you want to call it diaphragmatic breathing, abdominal breathing, deep breathing, stomach breathing, or belly breathing—learning to breathe correctly is the single most valuable daily practice you can do to enhance your health and well-being and prolong your life.

Reap the Rewards of Deep Breathing - Diaphragmatic breathing can be taught with simple breathing exercises. If you make a conscious effort to deepen your breathing, you'll reap the rewards of better sleep, you'll experience less fatigue, your mood will improve, and you'll have higher energy levels. Spend a few minutes twice a day on practicing breathwork.

Diaphragmatic Breathing Technique - Start by getting in a relaxed position, lying down with your knees bent. You may use a pillow or bolster roll underneath your knees. Focus on your breath for a few minutes as you breathe normally. Now place one hand on your upper chest and the other hand just below your rib cage on your abdomen. Take a deep breath, inhaling slowly and deeply through your nose, expanding your belly for seven seconds, then pause. The hand on your stomach should rise—the hand on your chest should move very little. Then exhale slowly through your mouth with pursed lips to a count of seven, contracting your abdomen, squeezing all the air out of your lungs.

Repeat this technique twice a day for 5-10 minutes or whenever you're feeling fatigued or stressed-out. Over time, and with a little practice, your breath will naturally become deeper, and your energy levels will soar.

35. Dry Skin Brushing: Health & Beauty Treatment

The skin is our largest organ of elimination. Our skin is responsible for 1/4 of our body's detoxification each and every day. Healthy skin should be eliminating approximately 2 lbs. of waste products per day. But, if the pores are clogged with millions of dead skin cells, then the toxins and impurities remain within the body.

Dry Brush for Gorgeous Skin & Glowing Health - The simple practice of dry skin brushing is one of the easiest and most powerful ways to help aid and enhance detoxification through the skin. Dry skin brushing has been practiced for centuries in many cultures, and is one of the simplest, yet most effective healing practices you can perform to keep your skin radiant, and your entire body healthy.

The Many Health Benefits of Dry Skin Brushing - It strengthens both the immune and nervous system, cleanses the lymphatic system, stimulates blood circulation, aids in digestion, tightens the skin, tones the muscles, breaks down and reduces cellulite, and gives you velvety soft, radiant skin.

How Do You Dry Brush? Dry skin brushing should be performed daily, before your shower or bath. Using a long handled natural bristle brush—start by brushing upwards from the soles of your feet up to your neck, in either long sweeping strokes or circular motions, always brushing towards your heart.

For Whole Body Health - Gently brushing the skin for just 5 minutes daily with a natural bristle brush, not only enhances the appearance of the skin by sloughing off old, dead, skin cells and helping new, healthy skin cells to regenerate—but this incredible anti-aging exfoliation treatment heals the whole entire body.

NOTE: DO NOT dry brush your face, and be gentle when brushing over the breasts, avoiding the nipple area.

36. Detoxify Your Body Naturally

If you suffer from low energy, chronic fatigue, frequent colds, allergies, headaches, indigestion, constipation, mood swings, anxiety, depression, and/or experiencing problems with your skin, it may be due to a build-up of toxins in your body.

Detox (short for detoxification) or otherwise known as an internal cleanse, is a very effective way to eliminate toxins from the blood, liver, kidneys, lungs, lymphatic system and the skin, while helping you achieve overall health. It's generally recommended to do a whole body cleanse at least once a year—not only to expel toxins, but to promote elimination, give the internal organs a rest, and refuel the body with healthy nutrients

Tips to Boost Your Health, Cleanse Your Body of Toxins, and Restore Internal Balance:

Upon awakening, takes a few minutes to stretch, and take several slow, deep breaths. By bringing more oxygen into the body, it promotes blood flow and lymphatic drainage, which is vital for removing toxins from the body.

Eliminate alcohol, caffeine, dairy products, salt, and refined sugar and flour during your detox. If you're a coffee drinker, opt for green tea instead. Green tea, which contains high levels of potent antioxidants, does contain some caffeine, but substantially less than coffee—and unlike coffee, the caffeine is released slowly into the system. Green tea boasts many anti-aging, health, and longevity benefits and has a positive impact on every system in the body including the cardiovascular, circulatory, respiratory, nervous, lymphatic, and immune.

Start out each day with a cup of warm lemon water. Just squeeze half a lemon into an 8 oz. glass of warm water. DO NOT use sugar! Warm lemon water stimulates the liver and aids in the digestion process while eliminating constipation.

Drink a minimum of 8 glasses of water daily to hydrate the body, flush out toxins, and restore health.

Eat 5-6 Small Healthy Meals Throughout the Day that Consists of:

- Fresh Organic Fruits and Vegetables

- Fresh Fish such as Salmon and Tuna

- Legumes and Beans

- Whole Grains

- Unsalted Nuts and Seeds

- Fresh Herbs and Spices

- Herbal Teas

NOTE: Eat NO processed foods! The more natural the diet, the better!

Take Your Supplements -Take nutrition and herbal supplements such as a full-spectrum, high potency multivitamin with minerals, omega-3 fatty acids, and milk thistle to enhance liver function.

Take a 30 Minute Walk Daily - Preferably outdoors to get some fresh air and a daily dose of vitamin-D from the sun. Exercise is an excellent way to rid your body of toxins through the skin, by sweating. Also, sitting in a sauna has the same effect.

Meditate - For 5-15 minutes daily to lower your stress levels. Meditation when practiced daily releases negative energy within your body and mind—as a result, this helps heal and enhance your physical, mental, emotional, and spiritual health. **NOTE:** For more information on the many health benefits of meditation—please refer to tip # 2.

Start Juicing - If you don't own a juicer, it's not required to go out and purchase one during a detox—but you may want to, as the health, healing, and anti-aging benefits of fresh juices are many. Besides providing more nutrition than sugar-laden store bought varieties, fresh homemade juices help to cleanse the body of toxins, boosts the immune system, and helps maintain the pH balance (making your body less acidic), while promoting health, healing, and energy.

How Often Should You Detox? The length of time a cleansing diet (or) detox is maintained, is based on your own individual needs. A cleanse can last from 1-10 days or more. Typically 3-5 days is sufficient time to reap the numerous rewards and benefits of detoxing. Many people opt to do a detox seasonally, others just once or twice a year. If you're not processing foods and eliminating waste properly, an internal cleanse may be just what your body craves.

NOTE: While detoxing, the first couple of days you may experience some mild side effects. Headaches are one of the most common, often due to caffeine withdrawal. Diarrhea, fatigue, or irritability may also be experienced while ridding the body of toxins. These side effects, while annoying, are actually a good thing, and usually pass quickly. Within a few days of detoxing, people often notice they have more energy, improved digestion, increased mental awareness, regular bowel movements, clearer skin, as well as an overall feeling of good health. Not to mention one of the best side effects of all... weight loss!

37. Sweat Your Way to Radiant Health

Most people know that sweating is our body's way of regulating our temperature. But did you know that sweating is an excellent way to expel toxins from the body? Sweating also improves circulation, relieves stress and fatigue, eases join pain and stiffness, provides pain relief, strengthens the cardiovascular system, lowers blood pressure, and promotes a healthy immune system. In addition, sweating burns calories for weight control, reduces cellulite, improves skin health, and induces better sleep.

Infrared Sauna Benefits - Infrared saunas, which are slightly different, and a lot more healing than normal saunas, have become increasingly popular. Infrared saunas make the same rays that come from the sun, but filters out the harmful UV rays. The health benefits of an Infrared sauna are numerous. They are an effective tool for detoxification, cardiovascular health, skin rejuvenation, pain relief, stress relief, as well as weight loss. You can actually burn up to 700 calories per session.

Bottom Line: Whether you sweat through exercise or through the use of a sauna, sweating has a huge impact on your overall health and quality of life. Learn to embrace sweating as a therapeutic method for promoting health, anti-aging, and well-being.

38. Chew More, Eat Less, Live Longer

When most people think of digestion, they often think of their stomach or intestines. The truth is, digestion starts in the mouth. The process of chewing is a vital component of the digestive process. If you're one of the many people who gulps down their food in a hurry, you may be setting yourself up for digestive problems such as heartburn, constipation, flatulence, stomach gas, bloating, and acid indigestion.

Chew Your Way to Better Health - When you chew your food slowly and thoroughly, your body releases powerful digestive enzymes in your saliva that help break down the food in your stomach. Chewing food properly and fully aids in the transport of nutrients to the body. This simple act helps convert the food into energy. When your food isn't digested properly, you can suffer from nutritional deficiencies and food sensitivities, as well as lethargy and low energy. Simply put, this means the vital nutrients in the food you're eating are being wasted, and your body isn't getting the nourishment it needs. Furthermore, undigested food particles can provoke bacterial growth in the intestines that can lead to health problems and possibly disease.

Added Bonus: Taking the time to chew your food properly (from 25-60 times, depending on the food you're eating), will help cut back on unwanted calories, and has the extra added benefit of weight loss.

39. Practice Emotional Freedom Technique (EFT Tapping)

Emotional Freedom Technique, also known as EFT tapping, is a powerful and life changing mind/body healing technique for relieving physical and emotional pain and discomfort. When our bodies are out of sync physically, mentally, or emotionally, this can trigger many health conditions, as well as illness. EFT can help restore the body's energy balance, so you can regain your sense of well-being.

EFT is sometimes called emotional acupressure, as it's similar to traditional acupuncture, but without the use of needles. By simply tapping on specific acupressure points with your fingertips, this powerful healing technique stimulates energy meridians in the body that help shift and release negative thought patterns or stressful emotions that hold us back in our personal lives, career, and relationships.

The List of Physical, Psychological, and Emotional Conditions for Which EFT is Used Are:

- Addictions

- Anger Issues

- Allergy Relief

- Abuse

- Attention Deficit Disorder (ADD – ADHD)

- Claustrophobia

- Depression

- Fears and Phobias

- Food Cravings

- Obsessive Compulsive Disorder (OCD)

- Pain Relief

- Stress

- Trauma

- Self-Esteem Issues

- Weight Loss

Key Point: Through the use of Emotional Freedom Technique, you can free yourself from negative feelings and beliefs, while dramatically transforming your life for the better, and adding quality years to your life.

40. Oxygenate With a Chi Machine

There are 3 things we cannot live without—food, water, and oxygen. We can live without food for weeks, (even months), without water for days, but only minutes without oxygen. Many of us suffer from lack of oxygen due to shallow breathing, a poor inadequate diet, lack of exercise, cigarette smoking, and/or air pollution. Oxygen starved cells in the body can result in low energy levels, shortness of breath, headaches, impaired mental clarity, chronic fatigue, sleep disorders, depression, intestinal problems, suppressed immune function, as well as many chronic diseases.

What is a Chi Machine? A chi machine is a passive exercise device that enables the body to gently rock from side to side (the same way a goldfish swims), maximizing the body's natural absorption of oxygen. The chi (meaning "life energy") creates a low-impact workout that requires no active movement, while getting the aerobic benefit equivalent of a 90 minute brisk walk (in terms of body oxygenation) in only 15 minutes.

The Primary Chi Machine Benefits Critical for Daily Cell Detox:

- Anti-Aging Health

- Oxygenates Every Cell in the Body

- Detoxifies - Ridding the Body of Toxins

- Weight Loss - Raises Metabolism Rate

- Aids in Maintaining Physical Wellness

- Aids in the Prevention of Illness

- Heals the Nervous System

- Increases Natural Energy - Greater Stamina

- Firms/Tones Hips, Thighs, Buttocks, and Abs

- Creates a Stronger Immune System

- Massages Internal Organs for Improved Function

- Aligns the Spine

- Reduces Back Pain & Improves Spinal Health

- Corrects Poor Posture

- Reduces Muscle Soreness, Tension, & Stiffness

- Creates Strong More Limber Joints

- Alleviates Many Stress Related Conditions

- Improves Blood Circulation

- Improves Digestive Health

- Stimulates Lymphatic Drainage

- Creates a Wonderful Sense of Well-Being

- Sounder More Restful Sleep

- Stimulates Alpha Brain - Wave Activity

- Enhances Mind/Body Healing

- Increases Libido

- Enhances Health and Longevity

- Maximizes the Body's Absorption of Oxygen

NOTE: A chi machine can be used by virtually everyone, even children, and is excellent for senior citizens, the physically impaired, bed-ridden, or frail.

Rebound - A mini trampoline, also known as a "rebounder," is also an excellent tool for oxygenating the cells and stimulating lymphatic drainage. **NOTE:** For more information on rebounding—please refer to tip # 57.

41. Color Therapy: Healing With Color

Color therapy has been around since the time of the Ancient Egyptians, when they discovered certain colors have a profound effect on the mind and body. Beautiful colors like red, blue, green, yellow, and orange can be used to enhance moods and emotions and reduce negative thought patterns by encouraging positive thought patterns to dominate.

There are 7 main energy centers in the body, which are referred to as chakras (sha kra). Color therapy is an alternative healing treatment that can be used to channel energy in positive directions through our chakras to improve our physical, mental, emotional, spiritual, and anti-aging health.

The Many Healing Properties of Color:

Red - The color red is associated with the base chakra. It promotes love, passion, and sexuality, as well as energy, stimulation, assertiveness and aggression. Red energizes the heart and the organs; therefore it is beneficial for people who suffer from fatigue and lethargy, and for those who could use a boost of self-confidence.

Orange - The color orange is associated with the spleen chakra. It promotes success, happiness, and sociability. Orange is extremely energizing. It stimulates creative

169

thinking, enthusiasm, optimism, and is a natural antidepressant. Orange can assist in healing conditions of the stomach and intestines, and is known to stimulate the lungs and thyroid gland to increase oxygen to the body.

Yellow - The color yellow is associated with the solar plexus chakra. It promotes cheerfulness, optimism, and wisdom. Yellow helps awaken inspiration and is uplifting for those who suffer from depression. Yellow is also an excellent color for nerve related conditions, as well as liver, stomach, and intestinal conditions.

Green - The color green is associated with the heart chakra. It promotes peace, balance, and harmony. Green induces a state of calmness and relaxation, stimulates growth hormone, and cures hormonal imbalances—and has also been found to be beneficial for those who have high blood pressure and cardiac conditions.

Blue - The color blue is associated with the throat chakra. It promotes communication, creativity, and personal expression. Blue cools and calms down inflammation, high blood pressure, and strong emotions, while strengthening and balancing the respiratory system.

Purple - The color purple is associated with the crown chakra located at the top of the head. Purple promotes creativity, spiritually, and intuition. Purple embodies both red (stimulating) and blue (calm). Purple has been found to be beneficial in the treatment of mental and nervous disorders.

NOTE: It's been shown that wearing bright, happy colors, as well as the colors we choose in our home, can be very therapeutic and significantly impact our moods. Wearing vibrant colored clothing can lift our spirits and can counteract feelings of depression, low self-esteem, and lack of confidence.

The 7 Chakras

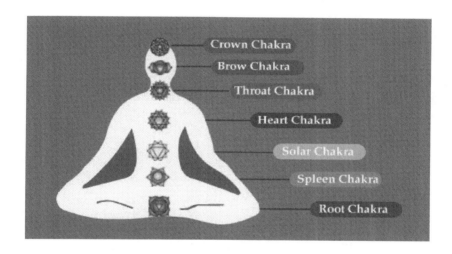

Crown Chakra
Brow Chakra
Throat Chakra
Heart Chakra
Solar Chakra
Spleen Chakra
Root Chakra

Part VI:

6 Tips That Will Make Your Libido Soar

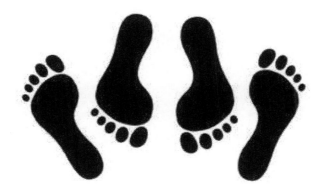

If you've reached middle age, and you're wondering where your sex drive has gone, you are not alone! Millions of women as they reach mid-life and enter into the perimenopause and menopause years notice a marked decrease in sexual interest. This is due primarily to an imbalance in the reproductive hormones estrogen and progesterone.

During menopause, levels of hormones decrease, leading to loss of libido. This is when many women report not only symptoms of low sex drive, but also vaginal dryness, hot flashes, depression, fatigue, weight gain, thinning hair, foggy thinking, and mood swings.

Causes of low sex drive can be physical or psychological. The important thing is to identify the reason for loss of libido. Only after this, can you find an effective solution and enjoy a healthy sex life again.

Often times, a few healthy lifestyle changes in combination with alternative treatments can help treat loss of libido, as well as other symptoms of menopause.

If you're one of the many women who suffer from sexual dysfunction due to hormonal changes...

Here are Some Tips to Help Rekindle Your Sexual Desire, While Helping You Feel More Youthfully Vibrant and Alive:

42. Eat a Libido Boosting Diet

Bad eating habits, along with a high-stress lifestyle, can really wreak havoc on a woman's hormones and can throw them out of balance. Symptoms of hormonal imbalance may include low sex drive, allergies, weight gain, depression, fatigue, facial hair growth, hair loss, and changes in the skin.

Diet plays a critical role in sexual function, including sex drive. To get your hormones back on track, add more lean protein to your diet and consume low-glycemic carbs rich in phytonutrients (plant-based foods), omega-3 essential fatty acids, as well as magnesium and zinc. Phytonutrients are naturally found in foods like fruits, vegetables, legumes, nuts, seeds, whole grains, and teas.

Feed Your Libido - Since chronic inflammation can exacerbate the symptoms of menopause and alter sex drive, it's recommended that you follow a libido boosting, anti-inflammatory diet, while lowering your intake of processed and refined foods. Eliminate all artificial sweeteners, and avoid foods that suppress sexual function and stress your adrenal glands, such as alcohol and caffeine. Also, limit starchy foods and sugar. And make sure to include a high quality multi-vitamin, a CoQ10 supplement, a calcium and magnesium supplement, and fish oil in your daily diet.

Natural Aphrodisiac Foods - Arouse or intensify sexual desire with these libido enhancing foods—chocolate (preferably dark), almonds, asparagus, avocado, bananas, caviar, cucumbers, figs, hemp seeds, honey, hot chili peppers, oysters, pumpkin seeds, wheat germ, and wine. Also, spices like cinnamon, cardamom, ginger, anise, garlic, basil, and turmeric have been known to enhance libido.

43. Balance Your Hormones Naturally

Our primary female sex hormones levels decline as we age. Women who suffer from menopausal-related symptoms including hot flashes, night sweats, mood swings, memory loss, vaginal dryness, decreased bone density, weight gain, and loss of libido, may benefit from the use of natural hormones.

Conventional hormone replacement therapy (HRT) is commonly prescribed for symptoms of menopause. Therapy can be given as a pill, patch, vaginal ring, skin gel, cream or spray. Hormone therapy has been shown to also reduce the risk of osteoporosis.

Bioidentical hormone replacement therapy (BHRT) is another treatment that has been used for years to help women experiencing these symptoms. Bioidentical hormones are identical to the hormones that are naturally produced by a woman's body. The primary goal of BHRT is not only to alleviate menopausal symptoms, but to restore hormonal balance to improve your quality of life.

For Optimal Health and to Naturally Keep Your Hormones in Balance:

- Consume a Healthy Diet

- Get Adequate Rest and Sleep

- Keep Stress Levels Low

- Exercise for 30 Minutes at Least 3 Times a Week

- Consume More Omega-3 Fatty Acids

- Take Hormone Balancing Herbal Supplements

- Avoid or Limit Caffeine and Alcohol

NOTE: If you are a woman who suffers from hormonal imbalance, it's recommended to consult a physician that specializes in female hormonal disorders, before using any type of HRT.

44. Herbal Remedies to Restore Low Sex Drive

There are two kinds of herbal supplements for treating loss of libido—phytoestrogenic herbs and non-estrogenic herbs. Phytoestrogenic herbs contain phytoestrogens, which produce compounds, similar to estrogen. These herbs are known to increase low estrogen levels. Non-estrogenic herbs do not contain estrogen, but instead are efficient at nourishing and balancing the hormonal glands.

Popular herbal supplements like horny goat weed, black cohosh, dong quai, wild yam, ginseng, maca root, and chaste berry are natural menopausal remedies that have been shown to increase sexual desire in women. The phytoestrogens and botanicals in these herbs have been used for centuries to help maintain healthy estrogen levels, while helping relieve the symptoms of menopause.

Herbal Menopausal Remedies That Have Been Shown to Increase Sexual Desire in Women:

Black Cohosh - Used as a folk remedy by Native Americans for a variety of female problems—black cohosh is a commonly used treatment of menopausal symptoms such as hot flashes (aka flushes), mood swings, irritability, vaginal dryness, lack of sexual interest, menstrual cramping, and sleep disturbances. Additionally, research indicates that black cohosh benefits in the reduction of inflammation symptoms of rheumatoid arthritis and osteoarthritis. Black cohosh is a common ingredient in most menopausal herbal combinations.

Chaste Berry - The chaste berry grows on the chaste tree, which is native to the Mediterranean region. Typically, the dried berries are used medicinally in capsules, tablets, tinctures, and teas. Chaste berry contains estrogen and progesterone like compounds, which regulate hormonal imbalance and counteract symptoms of menopause. Chaste berry may be combined with other herbs for maximum effect.

Dong Quai - A very popular herb in China where it has been used for thousands of years—dong quai, which is nicknamed the "female ginseng," alleviates vaginal dryness, reduces hot flashes, balances estrogen levels, increases sex drive, and regulates periods.

Ginseng - A part of Chinese medicine for more than 2,000 years—ginseng is a phytoestrogenic herb that contains human-like hormones, which increase estrogen levels in the body, and has been shown to help women who suffer from hormonal imbalance. Ginseng's benefits also include reducing symptoms of fuzzy thinking, inability to concentrate, and fatigue.

Maca Root - An extremely nutritious root—the maca root contains essential mineral and fatty acids and is rich in protein and vital nutrients. Maca root is extremely beneficial to women entering menopause, as it encourages and increases the balance between estrogen and progesterone. Maca root works well for symptoms such as hot flashes, night sweats, fatigue, mood swings, and loss of libido.

Red Clover - Red clover is a plant that is native to Europe and Asia. Used as a medicinal herb as a treatment for perimenopause and menopause—red clover contains isoflavones, which are plant-based chemicals that mimic the effects of estrogen on our bodies. These isoflavones help in managing the many physical and emotional symptoms of menopause. In addition, red clover is also an excellent source of nutrients.

Wild Yam - Used for centuries for the treatment of female problems such as menstrual cramps, menopausal, peri and post-menopausal symptoms—wild yam is considered a "natural alternative" for regulating the female system. Wild yam is used as an anti-inflammatory and hormone balancing herb and is available in cream form, as a supplement, as a tincture, and as a tea.

NOTE: Talk to your doctor or holistic prectitioner before using herbal medicine to treat menopausal symptoms.

45. Kegel Exercises for Better Sex

Kegel (pronounced KAY-gul) exercises were invented by Dr. Arnold Kegel to help women (and men, too) strengthen their pelvic floor muscles. Kegel exercises are often prescribed by doctors for new moms and women suffering from urinary incontinence. But, as an added bonus, studies show that by contracting and relaxing the muscles of the pelvic floor for 20 repetitions held for 3-5 seconds each, three times a day, on a daily basis—kegel exercises have been found to be one of the most effective ways to treat sexual dysfunction in women.

How are Kegal Exercises Performed? First empty your bladder. Pretend you are stopping the flow or urine. While isolating the muscles, squeeze or contract and hold for a count of 3-5 seconds, and then relax for 3-5 seconds and repeat. Start with 20 repetitions 3 times a day—and as you get stronger, build up to a minimum of 200 daily. It's important to breathe normally and use only the pelvic muscles. Kegel exercises can be performed lying on your back with your knees bent or can be done very inconspicuously anywhere or anytime—sitting at the computer, traffic lights, watching TV, etc. Consistency is key! Do kegel exercises daily and faithfully and you WILL see and feel the results!

46. Ignite Your Sex Life

We are all vital sexual creatures. Sexual activity has been called nature's fountain of youth. Sex raises the levels of life-extending hormones including endorphins, DHEA, and human growth hormones, while lowering stress hormones (cortisol), which can shorten your life span. Unfortunately, many people are missing out on the many health benefits of sex.

Many times in our hectic day to day lives, we just don't feel like it—and coupled with our loss of libido due to menopausal symptoms and hormonal imbalances, often time's sex is the last thing on our minds. But sex is part of the balance of life. Without sex, we're missing out not only on one of the great all-time pleasures in life, but on the numerous health and anti-aging benefits of having an active sex life for both women and men.

Get Hot and Healthy - Orgasms are natural stress relievers, releasing a cocktail of "feel good" hormones like oxytocin, endorphins (a natural opiate), serotonin, as well as DHEA into our body. Oxytocin is produced as a result of touch and is sometimes referred to as the "cuddle hormone," as it promotes feelings of affection. By increasing levels of DHEA into the body, it's proven to reverse aging by boosting the immune system and improving both brain function and cardiovascular health, as well as promoting younger, healthy-looking skin. Experts claim having sex generates estrogen, even during menopause, which may in turn, help to alleviate menopausal symptoms.

Get Your Groove Back - If you suffer from a loss of libido, there are ways to resurrect and rekindle your sexual desires. First, voice your concerns with your doctor. Get a complete exam, including a pelvic exam. Your doctor may look for physical and/or psychological causes that may cause loss of libido, such as prescription or over-the-counter medications, which can cause sexual dysfunction. By listening to your body and openly communicating with you doctor, you can get back to your old self and enjoy a healthy sex life once again. The worst thing you can do is ignore your symptoms and avoid having sex all together.

NOTE: For those who do not have a partner, there are other ways to achieve orgasm, such as through the use of adult toys and self-stimulation. Masturbation can be very empowering for women, as it gives you control over your body and sexuality, and is a great way to relieve sexual tension that can build up over time, especially for those without partners.

47. Aromatherapy for Menopausal Relief

The symptoms of menopause can significantly impact a woman's physical and emotional health and can lead to a decreased quality of life. Many women have turned to natural remedies to alleviate the symptoms of menopause, such as aromatherapy.

Aromatherapy is the practice of using the natural botanical oils extracted from the aromatic plants to enhance health and well-being. Essential oils are very powerful chemicals that influence hormone production, brain chemistry, and stress levels. Aromatherapy essential oils affect you physically, emotionally, psychologically, and spiritually and have been used for centuries for their antiseptic, anti-viral, antibacterial, and anti-fungal properties.

Aromatherapy Works in Two Ways - Through your sense of smell and absorbed through the skin. The inhaled aroma from essential oils is widely used to stimulate brain function. Suggested uses for essential oils are through inhalation, massage, with the use of a diffuser, and in the bath.

When it comes to alleviating menopausal symptoms, aromatherapy essential oils can have a remarkable effect on hormone balancing when combined with an effective diet and exercise plan—helping with both physical and emotional symptoms.

Ease Menopausal Symptoms With These Aromatherapy Essential Oils:

- **Hot Flashes** - Peppermint, Lemon, Clary Sage

- **Hormonal Imbalance** - Clary Sage, Fennel, Myrrh

- **Mood Swings** - Chamomile, Jasmine, Cypress

- **Fatigue** - Ginger, Peppermint, Pine Needle

- **Poor Memory** - Coriander, Ginger, Rosemary

- **Anxiety** - Chamomile, Jasmine, Lavender

- **Depression** - Bergamot, Neroli, Melissa

- **Irritability** - Patchouli, Cardamom, Neroli

- **Night Sweats** - Clary Sage, Basil, Thyme

- **Headaches** - Chamomile, Lavender, Peppermint

Combine a few drops of the essential oils with a few drops of a carrier oil (such as sweet almond), and massage into skin, or add 10 drops to your bath water and soak for 15-20 minutes.

NOTE: Before aromatherapy essential oils can be used, they must be diluted in a carrier oil since they are too potent to use alone. Carrier oils provide the necessary lubrication and 'slip and glide' to allow the hands to move freely over the skin and not drag while massaging. Carrier oils contain vitamins, minerals and essential fatty acids that moisturize and improve the condition of the skin.

Some of the Most Popular Varieties of Carrier Oils:

Acai Berry Oil - For all skin types—acai berry oil works well for mature, aging skin, as well as oily and acne prone skin. Rich in antioxidants and anti-inflammatory components, acai berry oil helps with skin conditions such as eczema and psoriasis.

Almond Oil (Sweet) - For all skin types—sweet almond oil is one of the most commonly used carrier oils. It works well for eczema and psoriasis, as it alleviates itching and calms inflammation. It's also good for sensitive and irritated skin.

Apricot Kernel Oil - For all skin types—apricot kernel oil is excellent for sensitive, delicate, or dehydrated mature skin and skin that is inflamed, irritated, or dry.

Avocado Oil - For dry, mature skin types—avocado oil nourishes and restores prematurely aged skin, severely dry, and sun damaged skin. Rich in vitamins and minerals and essential fatty acids, this extremely moisturizing oil has healing and regenerative properties.

Emu Oil - For normal, dry, mature, and sensitive skin— emu oil is an anti-inflammatory and is considered extremely healing. It's also helpful in reducing stretch marks, as well as conditions like arthritis and eczema.

Evening Primrose Oil - For all skin types—evening primrose oil works well for mature aging skin. Often taken internally as an herbal supplement, evening primrose carrier oil is used for PMS, menopausal symptoms, and rheumatoid arthritis. Evening primrose oil is also effective for treating acne and rosacea.

189

Flaxseed Oil - Suitable for dry skin—flaxseed oil is a valuable aid in scar healing, as it nourishes the skin and promotes cell regeneration. Flaxseed oil is also used to help treat eczema, psoriasis, acne, rosacea, and aging skin.

Grape Seed Oil - Good for normal, oily, and acne prone skin—grape seed oil is light in texture and high in antioxidants. And because grape seed oil is mildly astringent, it helps to tighten and tone the skin.

Hazel Nut Oil - For oily, combination, and acneic skin types—hazel nut oil encourages cell regeneration and has astringent properties, making it a very effective toner for the skin.

Hemp Seed Oil - For dry and aging skin—hemp seed oil is extremely high in essential fatty acids and aids in the reduction of wrinkles. Hemp seed oil is also widely used in the healing of inflammation of the skin and joints.

Jojoba Oil - For all skin types—jojoba is the number one carrier oil. Jojoba is actually a liquid wax that resembles sebum (the skins own natural oil). Jojoba also helps control oily skin and acne.

Maracuja Oil - For all skin types, but highly recommended for dry, mature, aging skin—maracuja oil, which comes from the passion flower, is a light oil, high in essential fatty acids and vitamin-C. Pure maracuja oil applied to the skin is non-greasy and can help assist in repairing, hydrating, soothing, and brightening dull, lifeless skin.

Olive Oil - Great for dry, cracked, aging skin—olive oil is a thicker oil, and should be blended with lighter carrier oil such as grapeseed. Used in many skin care and hair care products, olive oil is rich in fatty acids and anti-aging antioxidants.

Pomegranate Seed Oil - For all skin types—pomegranate seed oil works especially well for dry, mature skin. Pomegranate seed oil has been found to nourish the skin, reduce wrinkles, and improve skin's elasticity.

Rosehip Seed Oil - Great for normal to dry skin—rosehip seed oil works particularly well for aging skin, as this beauty oil has the ability to speed skin cell turnover, while promoting collagen and elastin production. Rosehip oil is also helpful in treating burns, sunburn, scars, and stretch marks.

Wheat Germ Oil - For dry, mature skin—wheat germ oil is helpful in the treatment of eczema, psoriasis, and prematurely aging skin. Wheat germ oil is a thicker oil and must be blended with a lighter oil.

WARNING! Wheat germ oil SHOULD NOT be used by people who have wheat allergies or gluten sensitivities.

Part VII:

10 Anti-Aging Tips That Have a Dramatic Impact on Your Skin's Health

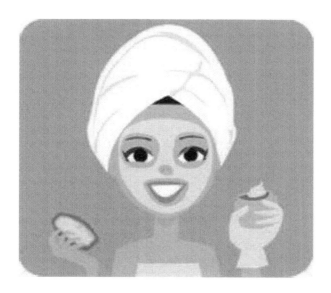

Your appearance is a pretty good indicator of the state of your health. Natural anti-aging skin care starts from the inside out. If you're experiencing problems with your skin, look at what you're putting into your body. Are you eating anti-aging foods high in powerful anti-aging antioxidants, like fresh fruits and vegetables? Are you drinking plenty of water and cutting back on refined sugar and white flour? Are you getting your omega-3 essential fatty acids (EFA'S) in supplement form, or better yet, in the foods you eat?

If you're not taking care of your internal health, it's going to show up externally. Chronic skin disorders like eczema, psoriasis, rosacea, and acne are all the result of your internal health.

Aging affects all of us. The first place we notice signs of aging is on our skin. Wrinkles, age spots, discoloration, and loss of elasticity are all tell-tale signs of aging. Fortunately, we can take steps to ensure younger, healthier, more vibrant skin. Thanks to new technology, there is a plethora of effective anti-aging skin care products on the market today to help combat the ravages of time on our skin.

With so many anti-aging skin care products on the market today, how do you choose? First and foremost, it's vital that you know your skin type. If you're unsure of your skin type, you can go online and get a personalized skin care evaluation. Once you've determined your skin type, consider special concerns you may have about your skin, such as age spots, dryness, fine lines and wrinkles, large pores, etc. Also, if you're sensitive to perfumes, dyes, and chemicals that are found in many skin care products, opt for an all-natural organic skin care line instead.

If you choose professional grade products, you are going to spend more than over the counter products, but when it comes to your skin, the investment is usually well worth it, when you see the results. Professional products contain stronger concentrations of AHA's, (alpha hydroxy acids) such as glycolic or lactic acid to help exfoliate dry, dead skin cells, and antioxidants such as vitamin-C and hyaluronic acid to moisturize, boost collagen and elastin production, and reduce fine lines and wrinkles.

These Skin Care Tips Will Have Your Skin Looking Years Younger and Healthier in No Time:

48. Avoid Excessive Sun Exposure

While you may think the look of tanned skin makes you look healthy, it's actually just the opposite. A tan is sun damage to the skin. The sun gives off ultraviolet radiation —UVA rays and UVB rays. UVB affects the outer layers of skin, while UVA rays are the more dangerous, and penetrates the deeper layers of skin. Excessive exposure to the sun is the number one cause of premature aging to the skin. Overtime, it can cause premature wrinkling, uneven skin pigmentation, or worse yet, skin cancer.

NOTE: Skin cancer is the most common type of cancer in the United States. Research shows that more than 3 million people are annually diagnosed with skin cancer. When you take into consideration that upwards of 10 thousand people die every year from skin cancer in the U.S. alone, you can see that healthy skin is really a matter of life and death.

Sensible Sunlight is Key - You hear so much about avoiding the sun to prevent cancer and wrinkles, but did you know that getting adequate safe sun exposure is key to vital health and is an important source of vitamin-D?!

Sunshine Deficiency - For years doctors told us the best way to prevent skin cancer was to avoid the sun as much as possible, and to slather sunscreen on our skin when we were exposed to the skin. That's all changed! For the past decade, experts have found that lack of sunlight and excessive use of sunscreens are responsible for the vitamin-D deficiency epidemic and higher cancer rates.

Sunshine Phobia - Our bodies get vitamin-D from sunshine, but unfortunately vitamin-D deficiency is becoming rampant due to our sunshine phobia. Vitamin-D, also known as the "sunshine vitamin" is one of the most underrated nutrients in the world! Vitamin-D has numerous immune system benefits, not to mention it's anti-aging benefits. This fat-soluble vitamin found in certain foods like salmon, eggs, and vitamin-D fortified milk, is also produced in the body when the skin is exposed to ultra-violet rays from the sun.

Soak Up the Sun's Energy - Unfortunately, studies show an epidemic level vitamin-D deficiencies from infancy to old age due to lack of sunlight. It's estimated that roughly 50% of Americans are deficient in vitamin-D; and then as we age, our ability to metabolize vitamin-D is reduced even more. Vitamin-D is not only anti-aging, but is essential for promoting calcium absorption, and is extremely energizing. Without sufficient vitamin-D, bones become thin, brittle, or misshapen.

Vitamin-D Deficiencies are Linked to:

- Increased Risk of Certain Cancers

- Autoimmune Disease

- Depression

- Osteoporosis

- Fibromyalgia

- Seasonal Affective Disorder (SAD)

- Muscle Weakness

- Chronic Muscle Pain

- Rickets in Children and Osteomalacia in Adults

Expose Yourself - Experts recommend getting 15-20 minutes of sunshine daily (before applying a sunblock), as the suns UV rays play an essential role in the production of vitamin-D. Soaking up just 20 minutes of sunshine a day, is a natural way to get your daily allotment of vitamin-D, while minimizing the risk of skin cancer.

Natural Alternatives to Chemical Sunscreens - While sunscreens may help to prevent sunburn, research shows that most commercial sunscreens contain toxic chemicals, which actually promote cancer. Chemical sunscreens block absorption of the ultra-violet radiation, which makes cancer fighting vitamin-D in the skin. Instead, opt for an all-natural biodegradable sunscreen lotion which contains no dangerous artificial chemicals and is actually healthy for the skin. Also, use an organic SPF lip balm to protect your lips from the sun.

How Often Should You Apply Sunscreen? Apply (natural) sunscreen every 4 hours and more frequently if you're in the water—and avoid or limit sun exposure during peak hours 10-2 pm. If it's unavoidable, wear UVA protective sunglasses and a sun visor or wide brimmed hat. Nowadays you can find a nice selection of sun protective clothing online and in stores.

What SPF Should You Use?

- For Fair Skin -Use an SPF of 30-50

- For Medium Skin - Use an SPF 15-30

- For Dark Skin - Use an SPF 8-15

When You Do Experience the Ravages of the Sun's Ultra-Violet (UV) Rays, These Natural Skin Care Remedies Can Provide Instant Pain and Itch Relief:

Milk Compress - Use cool compresses dipped in equal parts of cool water and whole milk and apply to the affected areas for 15-20 minutes; repeat every 2-4 hours. Rinse milk off so you don't smell sour! It's always best to use whole milk (not skim), as it's the fat in the milk that soothes the burn.

Aromatherapy Essential Oils - Add 15-20 drops each of lavender and chamomile essential oils to a tub of cool water and soak for 10-15 minutes. These healing aromatic essential oils help soothe the pain, reduce swelling and inflammation, and encourage skin repair.

Oatmeal Bath - Pour 1/2 cup of oatmeal into a tub of tepid water and soak for 15-20 minutes. Rinse and air dry. Oatmeal helps to avoid peeling and blistering.

Vinegar - Mix equal parts of apple cider vinegar and water and apply to affected area with a cotton ball. Or, put the vinegar/water concoction in a spray bottle and mist the sunburned areas. Vinegar will help prevent blistering and peeling. Let it dry and DO NOT rub!

Aloe Vera - While it's okay to use an aloe cream or ointment, it's best to use the plant itself. Break off a leaf from an aloe vera plant and rub the plants natural disinfecting gel onto the burn. Aloe vera is extremely healing and very effective in relieving pain, redness, itching, and inflammation.

Cucumber - Thinly slice fresh, cold cucumber lengthwise and place slices over the burn. Cucumber is very refreshing and soothing and relieves pain almost immediately, while reducing the redness. Cucumber works well for sensitive skin.

Tea - While most any kind of tea will help soothe the pain and itch associated with a sunburn—chamomile, green, black, white, peppermint, or spearmint work especially well! Tea can be used several different ways to relieve a sunburn. You can simply wet the tea bags and apply directly to the sunburned areas, or another option is to make a pot of tea, let it cool, and apply to the skin with a compress.

NOTE: In addition to being soothing sunburn remedies, these natural remedies for the skin also help alleviate the itching and irritation of eczema, psoriasis, as well as other inflammatory skin conditions.

Don't Overdo It! These skin care remedies help soothe a mild sunburn—but if you do overdo it and get too much sun exposure and you experience dizziness, fainting, nausea, fever, or chills—Immediately Seek Medical Attention!

Just Remember... Have Fun in the Sun, But Use Common Sense!

49. Use Cutting Edge Skin Care

Over time, as we age our skin incurs a lot of abuse! Cumulative sun exposure, biological factors, and environmental stresses all take its toll. Our skin becomes dull and less vibrant. In addition, you may be noticing fine lines and wrinkles, uneven pigmentation, blotchiness, age spots, and enlarged pores. Although these are all normal changes as we age, it doesn't mean we have to live with them!

The Good News is... Our skin is extremely resilient and responds well to TLC! By incorporating good quality anti-aging skin care products into your daily skin care regimen, you can dramatically fade skin discolorations, reduce wrinkles, and reduce visible signs of aging.

What's the Difference in Cosmetic Grade or Professional Quality Skin Care Products?

Whether you prefer to call it professional, pharmaceutical, dermatological, or medical grade—professional quality skin care products contain significantly higher strength formulas that deeply penetrate the skin. Cosmetic grade products are what you find in department, drug, and grocery stores and generally contain lower percentages of active ingredients—and some even contain synthetic chemicals that can actually be harmful to the skin.

Pharmaceutical quality is used only in professional grade products and is sold by Estheticians, Dermatologists, Medical Doctors, and Cosmetic Surgeons. A good quality anti-aging and/or anti-wrinkle treatment (botox alternative)** will contain significant levels of ingredients that will provide deep moisturization, while reducing fine lines, wrinkles, and expression lines. Pharmaceutical or professional grade anti-aging creams should also alleviate puffiness and darkening underneath the eyes, stimulate collagen and elastin production, and improve skin discolorations and age spots, while restoring your skins youthful appearance.

Botox Alternatives - There is so much hype these days about botox injections—but botox isn't for everyone! Especially if you're "needle phobic," or you have a fear of "face freeze." Luckily there are natural botox alternative, non-invasive skin care products popping up all over the place. Even though there is nothing quite as instantaneous as botox injections, these anti-aging wrinkle reducing skin care products offer effective results, and without the pain.

DO NOT Mix and Match Skin Care Products - Skin care manufacturers recommend using a skin care system from the same product line as they are created to work synergistically together. The active ingredients not only complement one another, but they're formulated with a specific pH balance. **NOTE:** The pH (potential of hydrogen) level refers to how acidic or alkaline your skin is. The amount of acid found in the skin determines the skin's resistance to bacteria. pH balance in the skin is a crucial part of what keeps our skin looking healthy and youthful. Applying a hodge-podge of different products that are not formulated to work together, can cause skin sensitivities, blemishes, rashes, and other irritations, and can throw the skin's natural pH balance off.

Anti-Wrinkle Cream Ingredients - The first thing you want to do when choosing an anti-aging wrinkle cream is to look at the list of ingredients. Look for an anti-wrinkle skin cream that contains ingredients like Copper Peptides, Alpha Hydroxy Acids, Retin-A Vitamin-C, and Vitamin-E. Also found to be beneficial in fighting signs of aging are CoQ10, Kojic Acid, Pycnogenol, and Green Tea. These are some of the top anti-aging ingredients that have been proven to significantly slow down and reverse visible signs of aging in skin.

What Do These Anti-Aging Ingredients Do For Your Skin?

Copper Peptides - Often referred to as one of the most effective anti-aging skin care ingredients, this facial rejuvenation treatment promotes skin firmness and density, stimulates collagen and elastin production, reduces photo-damage and hyperpigmentation, and is very healing to the skin.

Alpha Hydroxy Acid - Also known as AHA's—alpha hydroxy acids are made from fruit and milk sugars. The most common AHA's are glycolic acid (sugar cane), lactic acid (sour milk), malic acid (apples), citric acid (lemons and oranges), and tartaric acid (grapes). AHA's are very effective at exfoliating dry, dead skin cells, increasing collagen and elastin production, accelerating skin cell turnover and repair, reducing large pores, attracting moisture to the skin, reversing the effects of photoaging, and significantly reducing wrinkles. **NOTE:** Beta hydroxy acids (BHA's) such as salicylic acid are similar to alpha hydroxy acids, but are oil soluble, instead of water soluble, making BHA's a better choice for people with oily skin or acne.

205

Hyaluronic Acid - A natural substance found in abundance in young skin—hyaluronic acid is a highly effective humectant used in many skin care moisturizing products. This powerful hydrator reverses the signs of aging because of its ability to retain and hold moisture in the skin.

Retin-A - A form of vitamin-A—this powerful skin rejuvenator stimulates skin cell regeneration, builds collagen, diminishes age spots, reduces fine lines and wrinkles, reduces pore size, improves skin's hydration levels, improves skin's texture, and minimizes blemishes.

Vitamin-C - Also known as L-ascorbic acid—this powerful antioxidant protects the skin from inflammation, reverses and protects the skin against free radical and UV related damage, fades skin discoloration due to sun damage, tones and tightens the skin, boosts collagen production to help thicken the skin, and reduces fine lines, scars, and wrinkles.

Vitamin-E - An excellent moisturizer—vitamin-E is another antioxidant that has anti-inflammatory effects on the skin. Vitamin-E not only guards the skin against UV damage, but also reduces skin discoloration, age spots, and helps diminish scars and stretch marks.

CoQ10 - Found to be very beneficial in fighting signs of aging—CoQ10 reduces fine lines and wrinkles, repairs sun damaged skin, improves skin's elasticity and firmness, and diminishes the signs of photo-aging.

Kojic Acid - Found to have a similar effect as prescription strength hydroquinone—kojic acid is a natural skin lightener, which inhibits the production of melanin (brown pigment). Kojic acid works well for bleaching freckles, age spots, and skin conditions such as melasma (pregnancy mask).

Pycnogenol - A unique botanical extract—pycnogenol is one of the most powerful antioxidants on the market today. Pycnogenol increases skins elasticity and skin smoothness, which helps ward off wrinkles, while boosting hydration, and also helps dull skin look brighter and more luminous.

Green Tea - Gaining in popularity as a common ingredient found in natural skin care products—green tea is rich in antioxidants, which help prevent and protect the skin against sun damage. Green tea is also a powerful anti-inflammatory, and very soothing, and can help in the reduction of skin disorders like rosacea, eczema, and psoriasis.

Key Point: While we cannot stop the aging process, we can control the appearance of biological aging by helping our skin appear more youthful with the right anti-aging ingredients that deliver results, regardless of age.

50. Exfoliate Your Way to Radiant Skin

Exfoliation is an important part of skin care for both the face and body. Skin exfoliation is a great way to improve the look and health of our skin, especially as we age.

The skin is constantly renewing itself and shedding dead skin cells, at a rate of 30,000 - 40,000 per minute. The problem is, as our skin becomes mature, the process of skin cell turnover slows down significantly, leaving old, dead skin cells to accumulate on the surface of the skin, leaving the skin dull, dry, and flaky.

Exfoliation is beneficial to the skin because it dislodges the dead skin cells, revealing fresher, younger looking skin. Exfoliation also helps to unclog pores, allowing your moisturizer to penetrate deeper into the skin, while stimulating the regeneration of new, healthy cell growth.

Exfoliating can be done manually using a mildly abrasive scrub or exfoliating mask, and also through the use of chemical exfoliation, using fruit acids such as Alpha Hydroxy Acids (AHA's) or Beta Hydroxy Acids (BHA's).

NOTE: Hydroxy acids come in a variety of strengths ranging from 5-70%. While Estheticians are trained to administer glycolic peels containing 20-30% concentration, strengths above 35% should only be administered by a physician. Do your homework before using any type of fruit acid on your skin.

Less is More: Keep in mind, the goal of exfoliation is to leave your skin softer, smoother, and healthier, NOT red and irritated. When using a facial scrub, gently rub the scrub into damp skin, using a circular motion. It's recommended to exfoliate your face once or twice a week, and your body using a body scrub, up to 3 times a week. If you have extremely sensitive skin, you may want to exfoliate less often. After exfoliating, always follow up with a good moisturizer.

The One Exception - If you exfoliate your body with a natural bristle brush through the practice of dry skin brushing, this exfoliation procedure can (and should) be performed every day.

Alleviate Ingrown Hairs - Exfoliation may also help you avoid ingrown hairs after shaving or waxing, by preventing dead skin cells from plugging up hair follicles.

Advanced Method of Exfoliation - Microdermabrasion is a non-invasive skin resurfacing and rejuvenation treatment performed in day spas and dermatology clinics. Used on the face, hands, or neck—microdermabrasion sprays microscopic crystals over the skin's surface, removing the outer layer of dry, dead skin cells and revealing glowing, healthier skin underneath, while stimulating collagen and elastic production.

WARNING! Be sure to wear a (natural) sunblock of 15 or higher when out in the sun, as newly exfoliated skin tends to burn easily.

NOTE: For natural homemade facial and body scrub recipes—please refer to tip # 56.

51. Lighten & Brighten Your Skin

Everyone would like to have beautiful, clear, even-toned skin. But as we age, almost everyone of us suffers from skin discoloration, in one form or another. Uneven skin tone and/or hyperpigmentation can be the result of genetics, excessive sun exposure, hormonal imbalances, environmental factors, skin injury, or acne scarring. This can lead to sun damage, age spots (aka liver spots), melasma (pregnancy mask), freckles, and overall, a dull, lifeless complexion.

Skin lighteners and brighteners are a huge business. Sales continue to grow as baby boomers, who once worshipped the sun, are now relying on these products more than ever, to enhance both their facial and body skin.

What's the Difference in Skin Lighteners and Skin Brighteners? The main difference is that skin lightening formulas contain ingredients that penetrate the skin and decrease the amount of melanin (natural pigment) in the skin. Whereas, skin brighteners contain ingredients that do not change the skins function or structure, but enhance the skin by brightening and giving the skin a "glow," while improving skin tone and radiance with light-reflecting pigments.

Opt for Natural - Although historically, hydroquine was frequently used as a potent, medicinal skin lightening agent—all-natural skin lightening products nowadays typically rely on natural, yet powerful ingredients like kojic acid, mulberry extract, licorice extract, lemon extract, alpha-arbutin, glycolic acid, lactic acid, and vitamin-C to reduce the appearance of melasma, hyperpigmentation, and other skin discolorations.

Hydroquinone WARNING! While it's available over the counter in the United States, hydroquinone is a chemical bleaching (lightening) ingredient available in many skin lightening products. Do your homework before purchasing any products containing hydroquinone, as it's been banned by several countries for being a toxic chemical ingredient that is a potential carcinogen.

How Long Does it Take for Skin Lighters and Skin Brighteners to Work? It depends on the strength of the product and your own individual skin condition, but typically with daily use, you should see a noticeable difference in just 2-6 weeks.

The Good News is... Our skin is extremely resilient and responds well to TLC! By incorporating an anti-aging skin lightener or brightener into your daily skin care regimen, you can dramatically fade skin discolorations and reduce visible signs of aging.

NOTE: When using skin lighteners and/or brighteners, be sure to use a natural broad-spectrum sunscreen when in the sun, or the discoloration will just reappear.

52. Beauty Serum: The Magic Skin Elixir

Anti-aging skin care products is a multi-billion dollar industry that is growing every day. In the quest for healthier, younger, more youthful looking skin—beauty serums have become one of the hottest skin care products around. Used for years in spa's as part of a facial treatment, beauty serums are generally water or oil based, and because they have a smaller molecular structure, penetrate the skin deeper than a cream.

Serums Many Anti-Aging Benefits - Look for serums that contain high levels of antioxidants like vitamins A, C, and E. These age reversing antioxidants destroy free radicals, prevent and repair damaged skin, reduce fine lines and wrinkles, stimulate collagen and elastin production, and hydrate and firm sagging skin.

How to Apply Facial Serum - Serums tend to be a bit pricey, but are highly concentrated, so you use less, so they will last longer. As part of a daily skin care regimen, they're generally applied once or twice a day, after the toner, and before the moisturizer. And because damp skin is 10 times more permeable than dry skin, apply the serum right after the toner, while the skin is still moist, to boost effectiveness and to assure deeper penetration of the active ingredients. Once the serum is completely dry, then apply your moisturizer.

53. Mask Your Imperfections

The many benefits of anti-aging facial masks (or masques) have been known for centuries. Facial masks can be applied as a cream, clay, or gel. Other popular masks are the peel-off mask and the sheet mask which is a soft, very thin piece of cloth. Using a facial mask just once a week can vastly improve the health and beauty of your skin. However, it's okay to use a mask a couple of times a week, depending on your skin type and the type of mask you are using.

There are Many Different Kinds of Facial Masks for Different Purposes:

- **Deep Cleansing** - For All Skin Types

- **Clay (Mud)** - For Oily & Combination Skin

- **Collagen** - For Mature Skin

- **Hydrating** - For Dry & Mature Skin

- **Firming** - For Mature Skin

- **Enzyme** - For All Skin Types

- **Exfoliating** - For All Skin Types & Dull Skin

- **Self-Heating** - For All Skin Types

- **Skin Brightening** - For All Skin Types

- **Water Based Gel** - For Sensitive Skin & Rosacea

Facial Mask Benefits: No matter what your skin type, there is a facial mask for you. Facial masks contain high concentrations of ingredients to deep clean, oxygenate, and nourish the skin. The other benefits include drawing out bacteria and toxins, tightening pores, exfoliating, brightening, and hydrating the skin.

NOTE: For natural homemade facial mask recipe— please refer to tip # 56.

216

54. Replenish Lost Moisture

While different skin types have different needs, one thing all skin types (even oily) have in common, is the need for moisture. Moisturizing the skin is extremely important for keeping the skin properly hydrated, healthy, and supple, and the skin barrier strong. Especially as we age, a good anti-aging moisturizer is an absolute beauty essential!

Aging Skin Loses Moisture - When we are young, our skin contains ample amounts of hyaluronic acid. Hyaluronic acid (also known as HA), is produced naturally in the cells and tissues of the body. HA helps to keep skin hydrated and plumped, as it attracts water and has the ability to hold up to thousand times its weight in water. As we age, our hyaluronic acid levels diminish significantly. Fortunately, HA is a key ingredient found in many moisturizers and skin care products. When used in skin care, HA dramatically improves skin's hydration.

If You're Over 40... A good rule of thumb when picking an anti-aging moisturizer, is to look for one that contains an SPF of at least 15. Also, choose a product that contains high levels of antioxidants to protect your skin from free radicals, while strengthening the skin. Choose natural skin care products over products that contain harsh chemicals and perfumey scents, and apply your moisturizer daily, but don't overdo it, to avoid clogging pores!

55. Consistency with Skin Care is Key

The enemy of beautiful, radiant skin is not so much aging, as it is damage to our skin. 80% of visible aging is a result of individual lifestyle, diet, personal hygiene, and our environment. The anti-aging secret to achieving truly beautiful, healthy skin lies in not covering up the problem, it lies in using anti-aging skin care products that deeply penetrate the layers of skin to repair, protect, and restore the natural skin barrier.

Make the Commitment - Healthy skin starts with a commitment to a regular skin care regimen using good quality skin care products. It's important to cleanse, tone, and moisturize on a daily basis, then exfoliate once or twice a week with a mild scrub. For an added treat, pamper yourself with a beauty mask for your particular skin type, but refrain from using a facial mask more than once or twice a week, unless the directions on the mask say it's okay.

Choosing an Eye Treatment - As we age, the eyes are one of the first places to show signs of aging. Eye creams and serums target the delicate eye area and help to alleviate the many signs of aging by lifting and tightening sagging skin, diminishing fine lines, wrinkles, and crow's feet, and minimizing the appearance of dark circles and puffiness. Because the skin around the eye area is more delicate, always apply a cream or gel with your ring finger, as this is the weakest finger and it won't stretch the skin, which may lead to premature wrinkling.

NOTE: Eye creams and serums contain more oil than facial lotions, because the skin around the eyes have fewer oil glands and tend to be dryer than the rest of the face.

Don't Neglect the Skin Below Your Chin - When we think of skin care, we generally think of the skin on our face. The skin on our body needs attention too! Prevent dry, itchy skin by using a good body lotion to moisturize. And don't forget to dry brush on a daily basis and use a body scrub to exfoliate two to three times a week. Pay special attention to your knees, elbows, and feet as these areas are often times the most neglected parts of the body. Using a pumice stone daily during your shower or bath can help soften and reduce rough, callused skin on the soles and heels of the feet. This can also work wonders in helping to lighten and smooth the dark, dry skin on the knees and elbows. Always follow up with a rich emollient cream or lotion designed to repair extra dry skin.

Get Your Beauty Sleep - For radiant skin, make sure you get plenty of sleep. Skin repairs itself while we sleep, so if you're chronically sleep-deprived, your complexion will show it. Remember to always apply a night cream or serum before bed, and protect your skin during the day with a good (natural) sunscreen SPF 15 or higher.

Key Point: Proper skin care helps protect skin from the aging process and helps reverse some of the damage already done. Giving your skin the nutrients it needs is vital in helping your skin look young, healthy, and vibrant. Pamper your skin and it will age more slowly!

56. Natural Homemade Skin Care Recipes

There's nothing better than treating yourself to a little pampering with a professional spa facial! But in these rough economic times, it's not always affordable or practical. To help maintain healthy radiant skin between professional treatments... Do It Yourself!

Many of us don't realize that we can whip up our own holistic, natural skin care treatments with ingredients found in our own kitchens. Homemade beauty treatments are a fun and economical way to create an indulgent spa-like facial at home. Containing natural ingredients, these homemade skin care recipes have a powerful impact on the health and appearance of the skin! Using organic ingredients are preferable, but not necessary to achieve beautiful, glowing skin.

PLEASE NOTE: The following recipes are intended for a single application and can be used once or twice a week. Make sure your skin is properly cleansed and completely dry first, before applying a mask. Use a clean fan brush or small paint brush, or simply apply with your fingertips in a circular motion, spreading a thin layer over the entire face and neck area. Leave the mask on for 15-20 minutes, then rinse off using warm water and a washcloth. Next, apply a facial toner with a cotton ball to ensure there are no traces of the mask remaining on the face. Follow up treatments with your favorite moisturizer.

FOR DRY and AGING SKIN:

Whether your skin concerns are age spots, fine lines and wrinkles, dryness, sagging skin, or a combination...

Here are some easy anti-aging skin care recipes that will help prevent and reverse signs of aging, while helping your aging skin look healthy and radiant!

Banana Anti-Aging Mask

1 Small Ripe Banana
1 Tbsp. Honey
2 Tbsp. Milk (whole milk preferably)

Mash banana until creamy, add milk and honey; mix well. Apply to face and throat. Leave on for 20 minutes. Rinse with warm water, followed by a cool rinse.

Avocado Hydrating Anti-Aging Facial Mask

1/2 Avocado (peeled and mashed)
1/4 C. Milk (whole milk preferably)
1 Egg White - beat until stiff.

Mix ingredients into a smooth paste. Apply to face and throat. Leave on for 20 minutes. Rinse with warm water, followed by a cool rinse.

Cucumber Anti-Wrinkle Peel

1/4 Cucumber (peeled and seeded)
1 Egg White (beaten)
1 tsp. Lemon Juice (fresh)

Puree ingredients in a blender. Apply to face and throat. Leave on the skin for 20 minutes. Rinse with warm water, followed by a cool rinse.

Anti-Aging Skin Firming Facial

1/2 tsp. Vitamin-E Oil
2 Tbsp. Plain Yogurt
1 Egg (beaten)

Mix ingredients and apply to face and throat. Leave on for 20 minutes. Rinse with warm water, followed by a cool rinse.

Anti-Aging Moisturizing Body Lotion

1 Tbsp. Honey
1 tsp. Extra-Virgin Olive Oil
1/2 tsp. Fresh Lemon Juice

Mix well and massage into dry patches on elbows and knees. Leave on for 20 minutes. Wash off with warm water.

FOR OILY and ACNE PRONE SKIN:

Strawberry - Honey Acne Mask

1/2 C. Fresh Strawberries
1 Egg White
2 tsp. Honey

Puree ingredients in a blender. Apply to face and throat. Leave on the skin for 20 minutes. Rinse with warm water, followed by a cool rinse.

Honey - Apple Mask

1 Medium Apple (grated into a fine pulp)
3-4 Tbsp. Honey

Mix ingredients and apply to face and throat. Leave on for 20 minutes. Rinse with warm water, followed by a cool rinse.

Apple Cider Vinegar Skin Toner

2 Tbsp. Apple Cider
1 Cup Pure Spring Water

Mix ingredients in a glass jar. Soak a cotton ball with toner and gently rub over the face, leaving solution on the face. DO NOT rinse off. Use 1-3 times daily for acneic skin. Will last up to 2-3 months in the refrigerator. **NOTE:** Undiluted apple cider vinegar can also be also be dabbed on pimples as a spot treatment.

FOR SENSITIVE SKIN:

Cucumber - Aloe Facial Mask

1/4 Cucumber (peeled and seeded)
2 Tbsp. Pure Aloe Vera Gel
1 Tbsp. Plain Yogurt

Puree cucumber in blender. Mix in remaining ingredients and apply to face and throat. Leave on for 20 minutes. Rinse with warm water, followed by a cool rinse.

Sensitive Skin Exfoliant

2 tsp. Baking Soda
1 T. Extra-Virgin Olive Oil
2-3 Tbsp. Milk (preferably whole milk)

Mix ingredients and gently massage into the skin in a circular motion. Rinse with warm water, followed by a cool rinse.

FOR ALL SKIN TYPES:

Pumpkin Enzyme Brightening Mask

1 Tbsp. Pumpkin Puree (canned without spices)
1 tsp. Honey
1 tsp. Milk (preferably whole milk)

Mix ingredients and gently massage into the skin in a circular motion. Rest or relax for 20 minutes. Rinse with warm water, followed by a cool rinse. **NOTE:** This mask works well for all skin types, but works especially well for dull looking skin.

Brown Sugar Body Scrub

2 Tbsp. Brown Sugar
2 Tbsp. Oatmeal (uncooked)
1 Tbsp. Honey
1 tsp. Lemon Juice (freshly squeezed)
1 Tbsp. Extra-Virgin Olive Oil

Grind oatmeal in a blender or food processor until ground very fine. Mix all ingredients into a paste. Use in the shower while skin is moist. Massage in a circular motion with a wash cloth. Rinse off with warm water. (This scrub can also be used on the face and lips).

Green Tea Toner

1 Green Tea Bag
1 Cup Pure Spring Water

Make 1 Cup of green tea, let steep for 10 minutes. Remove tea bag and let cool to room temperature. Mix with pure spring water. May store in glass jar or spray bottle. Soak cotton ball with mixture and apply to the face or lightly mist with spray bottle. Will last in refrigerator for up to 1 week.

Natural Ingredients Skin Care Benefits:

Apple - Containing malic acid and powerful antioxidants –apples are a gentle exfoliant.

Apple Cider Vinegar - Detoxifying and healing—raw unfiltered apple cider vinegar restores skin's natural pH balance and helps absorb excess oil from the skin.

Aloe Vera - Rich in over 200 nutrients—aloe vera is soothing, healing, moisturizing, and firming.

Avocado - Rich in potent antioxidants, vitamins, and minerals—avocado is excellent for dry, aging skin.

Baking Soda - Aids in cleansing—baking soda is an inexpensive and effective gentle exfoliation treatment.

Banana - High in potassium and vitamins—bananas nourish, soften, and moisturize the skin.

Eggs - High in protein—egg whites give skin a lifting and tightening effect and helps reduce large pores.

Honey - Anti-fungal and anti-bacterial—raw honey (especially manuka honey) is rich in vitamins and minerals and soothes, softens, tones, and heals skin.

Lemon - Anti-wrinkle, anti-bacterial, antioxidant, and antiseptic—lemon is a natural skin brightener. Diluted lemon juice is also an effective toner for acne-prone skin.

Milk - Containing lactic acid—milk gently exfoliates, soothes, moisturizes, and softens skin.

Extra Virgin Olive Oil - Rich in antioxidants and fatty acids—EVOO is nourishing, soothing, and extremely moisturizing.

Pumpkin - Excellent source of anti-aging antioxidants—pumpkin promotes skin repair, exfoliation, and hydrates.

Sugar - A gentle exfoliant, rich in natural glycolic acid—sugar promotes cellular renewal.

Strawberries - Rich in salicylic acid—strawberries gently exfoliate dead skin cells, removing impurities, while helping make pores appear smaller.

Yogurt - A natural skin moisturizer—yogurt is a gentle cleanser and exfoliant that gives skin a beautiful glow. Yogurt also reduces pore size and improves skin's texture, while restoring skin's natural pH balance.

NOTE: 2 tsps. of Baking Soda may be added to any of the facial mask recipes or your commercial skin care products to further enhance gentle exfoliation.

57. Diminish Cellulite Naturally

Cellulite ranks right up there with wrinkles and gray hair, as one of most unwelcome signs of aging. In the quest to get rid of cellulite, women have tried everything from cellulite reducing creams to costly cosmetic treatments like Endermologie or VelaShape. While these treatments have shown some promising results, a low-fat diet and regular low-impact aerobic exercise turns out to be one of the most effective therapies, and the healthiest.

Practically every woman, whether she's overweight or not, will have some degree of cellulite in her lifetime. The female hormone estrogen is to thank for that. Genetics can play a key role, as well as poor circulation, lack of oxygen in the cells, and bad eating habits. In addition, as we age our skin tends to lose some of its elasticity, especially for those who don't exercise. Regular exercise stimulates lymphatic drainage, while toning the muscles underneath the skin, which keeps skin taut and ripples at bay.

Luckily There are Some Amazing Anti Cellulite Treatments and Remedies That Really Work!

Coffee Scrub - Take coffee grounds from your morning coffee, mix in 2 tablespoons olive oil, a dash of both cayenne pepper and cinnamon, and 1 tablespoon of honey. While in the shower, using a loofah or massage glove, massage the mixture in a circular motion over your buttocks and thighs for a few minutes, then rinse off. The caffeine in the coffee tightens the skin, the coffee grounds promote circulation, the cayenne pepper and cinnamon draw blood to the surface to further promote blood circulation, while the honey naturally moisturizes the skin and keeps it supple.

Bounce Away Cellulite - Mini trampoline jumping also known as "rebounding" is one of the best exercises you can do for getting rid of cellulite. Rebounding consists of jumping up and down and jogging in place on a mini trampoline, otherwise known as a rebounder. Just rebounding for 10-20 minutes a day, is an excellent way to reduce cellulite, while burning fat and calories and lifting, tightening, and toning your hips, legs, butt, and stomach.

NOTE: When you bounce on a rebounder, it stimulates the lymphatic system, which helps to flush out toxins and waste. Many women report seeing significant improvement in their cellulite in as little as two weeks.

Daily Massage - Massage cellulite prone areas daily with an essential oil blend of juniper, rosemary, lavender, and cypress diluted with sweet almond carrier oil. This blend helps stimulate circulation, while removing fat and toxins.

Dry Skin Brushing - This simple, yet very effective technique helps improve the appearance of cellulite by stimulating blood and lymph flow, eliminating toxins, exfoliating the skin, and encouraging new cell growth. By gently brushing cellulite-prone areas with a natural bristle brush every day, this helps to break up fat deposits and improve the overall health of your skin. **NOTE:** For more information on dry skin brushing—please refer to tip # 35.

Tweak Your Diet - Reduce sodium (salt) intake, eliminate artificial sweeteners and food additives, fried foods, and junk food, and make extra virgin olive oil a part of your daily nutrition.

Drink Cranberry Juice to Fight Cellulite - Cranberries are a potent source of antioxidants and bioflavonoids, and can work wonders for helping eliminate cellulite. Mix 1 oz. 100% unsweetened cranberry juice with 1 cup water and sip throughout the day. This cellulite reducing concoction helps cleanse and emulsify fat in the lymphatic system, detoxifies the liver, improves blood circulation, and helps eliminate water retention. By drinking just 4 cups a day of this cranberry-water mixture, you should start seeing an improvement in your cellulite in as little as 2-3 weeks.

Bikram Yoga - Performed in a 100-110 degree yoga studio, bikram yoga is extremely detoxifying as it makes you sweat like no other, as you perform 90 minutes of 26 yoga poses. **NOTE:** For more information on bikram yoga –please refer to tip # 5.

WARNING! Consult with your doctor before starting Bikram yoga, especially if you are a beginner.

Part VIII:

20 Anti-Aging Tips That Promote Peace, Harmony, and Longevity

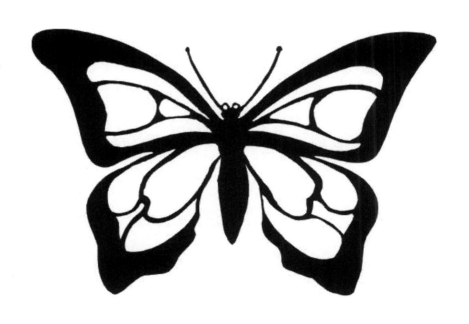

Jugglers make it look so easy, tossing one ball after another up into the air—but juggling work, family, and life's responsibilities, isn't always as easy. Trying to find balance in our fast-paced, hectic lives can leave us feeling stressed, overwhelmed, and emotionally taxed. This can wreak havoc on our bodies, minds, and spirits and can lead to premature aging, as well as weakening our immune systems and setting ourselves up for ill health.

Being true to ourselves, finding more pleasure in simple things, having a close-knit group of friends and family, and living our lives in balance can add many happy years to our lives.

The Following Tips Have an Extremely Positive Impact on Your Mental, Emotional, and Spiritual Health:

58. Be True to Yourself

Being true to you is all about being your authentic self, embracing and accepting yourself, imperfections and all. Learning to love yourself is the first step. How do you expect others to love you, if you don't love yourself? Self-love is not about having a big ego or being conceited, it's about feeling good about yourself, your strengths, and your accomplishments. It's about valuing the person you truly are.

Just Be Yourself - Many people wander through life, never really knowing their true authentic selves or their potential. Be honest with yourself—be open about your wants, your needs, your desires, and your goals. Just be yourself. We all have the capabilities to be generous or selfish, loving or hateful. It's up to us to choose which characteristics we want to nurture or not.

Stop Judging - We live in a highly judgemental society. We judge our friends, neighbors, co-workers, celebrities, politicians, and even random people around us. More so than that, we judge ourselves. Judging ourselves and others can only foster negativity. We must move beyond that and be more accepting of ourselves and other people.

Embrace Your Imperfections - None of us are perfect, nor should we want to be. Learn to be comfortable in your skin, flaws and all. If your flaws are holding you back from personal growth, work on them. But, don't try to be someone you're not, or compare yourself to others. We've all got certain things we like and don't like about ourselves. Focus on your personal attributes and celebrate your uniqueness. Be genuine, follow your heart, and your passions, and listen to your inner-voice. Think positive, believe in yourself, and stand up for what you believe in.

59. Create Balance in Your Life

Sometimes we get so caught up in our busy day to day lives, that our lives literally spin out of control, leaving us feeling totally out of balance. The key to achieving a well-balanced life is about prioritizing. It's about integrating and aligning the most important components in our lives.

Create a Pie Chart of Your Life - This a great visual tool that may help get your life in balance. Section off the various areas of your life like: family, work, health and fitness, social life, recreation, hobbies, God, spiritual growth, etc. This way you can visually see if your life priorities are being met. Next, make a second chart with how you want your life to be. Now you can focus on what changes need to be made to realign your life and get your life in balance.

Life is a Balancing Act - If you're working too much, or putting too much focus on certain areas of your life, and ignoring others, it will eventually catch up with you. Make it a point to schedule time with family and friends and make time for activities that nurture you and help you recharge.

Restore Harmony - Finding balance can reduce stress while restoring harmony in your life. If your life is out of balance, examine your priorities and make the necessary changes. Help restore your body's natural healing potential by taking the time and effort to focus on the things in life that bring you fulfillment and happiness.

Life Balance Wheel

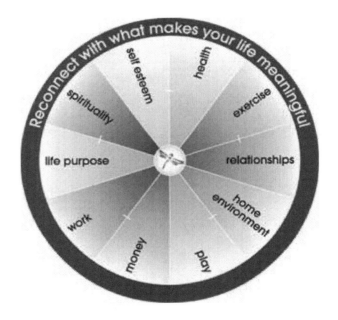

60. Find Pleasure Daily

There are the universal pleasures like food, sex, and companionship. But for the most part, we are not really experiencing as much pleasure as we could be in our daily lives. We live in a fast-paced society, where we're all moving at warp-speed, with ridiculously long to-do lists. We need to re-learn to connect with ourselves and others. It's important to find some time every day to search for things that bring us sheer joy and pleasure. That goes hand in hand with being present in our lives, and mindfully paying attention to what's going on around us.

Pleasure Awakens the Senses - What makes you smile? What brings you joy or stirs feelings of passion? Renew your sense of wonder. Tap into that sense of wonder you had as a child.

Add Music to Your Daily Life - Music is one of our greatest all-time pleasures. While most of us enjoy listening to music—did you know that music affects our thoughts, feelings, and behaviors? Research shows that music has a profound impact on our health and psyche. Music can be relaxing or energizing, and can deeply affect us physically and emotionally. Listening to our favorite songs boosts our brain health, while reducing stress, anxiety, chronic pain, and depression.

Music is Food for the Soul... A daily dose of your favorite music is not only extremely pleasurable, but can boost your immune system, resulting in less illness, and can add years to your life.

Bottom Line: Reconnect with the people and things that give you pleasure, enjoyment, and meaning, and live your life with zest and gusto! Shed those nagging feelings of pessimism. Be kind to yourself and others, and make a decision to live with joy, happiness, and optimism.

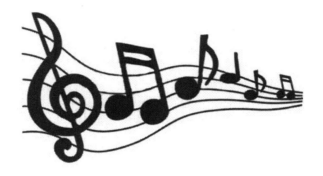

61. Make Self-Care a Top Priority

Self-care is all about personal care maintenance—making time for ourselves—mind, body, and spirit. How well we treat ourselves reflects on our overall health and well-being, not to mention—our life span. Self-care is not about self-indulgence—self-care is about choosing positive, self-compassionate, self-nurturing behaviors that balance our physical, mental, emotional, and spiritual well-being.

Implement Self-Care Into Your Life - Self-care starts with taking care of our physical selves—our teeth, hair, and skin, as well as a daily routine of eating healthy foods, getting proper rest, getting exercise, practicing meditation, abstaining from substance abuse, and pursuing creative outlets. A well-nourished mind, body, and spirit is vital for high self-esteem, emotional balance, consistent energy, and overall enjoyment of life.

Don't Slack Off When it Comes to Your Appearance - Many times in our busy fast-paced lives, we don't take (or make) the time to make our physical self-care a top priority. Every aspect of our appearance, as well as our personal hygiene and grooming, shows the world what and who we are. Feeling good about our appearance comes from within. Having a well-cared for body not only makes you feel good and projects confidence, but conveys to others that you value and respect yourself.

Smile More to Improve Health and Attractiveness -
We are naturally drawn to people who smile. People who
smile exude confidence. Smiling naturally releases endorphins, boosts the immune system, lowers blood pressure, and relieves stress.

A Good Reason to Whiten Your Smile - If you want to
take years off your appearance—whiten and brighten
your teeth. As we age, the enamel on our teeth becomes
thinner and more transparent, causing the teeth to look
darker. A dazzling smile not only makes you look more
attractive, but can make you look and feel years younger,
more vibrant, and more confident.

Don't Forget to Pamper Yourself - Take some well-
deserved time to rest, relax, and rejuvenate your mind,
body, and soul. Treat yourself to a spa day or a relaxing
massage. But don't wait for a special occasion to pamper
yourself—take some time for yourself every day.

Bottom Line: Improve your physical, mental, and emotional health by taking responsibility for your own well-being and by making choices to promote self-care.

62. Listen to Your Body and Soul

Listening to your body's internal messages is vital for maintaining good health and anti-aging. Sometimes we lose connection with the most fundamental signals of life, the internal information that speaks to us through various bodily sensations and emotions. It's time to wake up and become conscious of not only our body, but our mind and spirit, as well. It's all about learning to pay attention and using awareness and deep intuition to make smart choices about our health and well-being.

Are You Really Listening? How often do you ignore your body's basic needs? Do you eat when you are hungry, and stop eating when you've had enough? Do you get as much sleep as you need or rest when you are tired? How often do you listen to your gut instinct? Our body sends out cues—some subtle, others are loud and practically scream at us.

Tap Into Your Intuition - If you're not in tune with your body, it may take some practice at first, but if your health and happiness is a priority, it's vital to listen to, and honor your body's needs. By taking the time to focus and really pay close attention to what your body, as well as your intuition is trying to tell you—you will become more connected and balanced in all aspects of your life.

How Well Do You Really Know Yourself? It's a question many of us struggle with. Knowing yourself means knowing your interests, behaviors, qualities, passions,

243

values, beliefs, hopes, fears, strengths, weaknesses, tolerances, limitations, idiosyncrasies, and your purpose in life. It seems like a no-brainer—after all, who spends more time with ourselves than we do? But truly knowing ourselves can be difficult and takes a conscious effort.

Observe Yourself - Start by observing yourself and your behavior as objectively as possible—as if you're seeing yourself through the eyes of other people—like looking in a mirror. Self-observation prompts you to pay closer attention and to be more aware of your thoughts, feelings, behaviors, and reactions.

Make a List - Write down all the things you know best about yourself—your likes and dislikes, your interests and passions, your unique gifts and talents, your dreams and goals, etc. Creating a list of your personal attributes (positive and negative) is an important aspect in the process of discovering your own individuality.

Keep a Personal Journal - Journaling is a great way to chronicle your day and to get to know yourself better. Writing down your thoughts, feelings, ideas, and desires is not only cathartic, but is a wonderful tool for self-discovery and self-realization.

Personality Quiz's - The internet is a great place to find hundreds of free personality tests and quizzes. By taking these tests, you can discover your personality type, along with some important facets of your personality.

Bottom Line: As you begin your journey to self-discovery and growing self-knowledge, you'll grow more and more in touch with yourself. You'll likely find that you're able to make better decisions, you'll make more positive lifestyle choices, and ultimately find more meaning and purpose in life.

63. Discover Your Life's Calling

According to a recent survey, roughly 75% of people do not know what their true calling is. Whether you call it your life's purpose or your life's calling, each and every one of us is a unique individual with certain talents and gifts. Unfortunately, most people meander through life never really discovering their life's calling. If you're at a crossroads and don't know which way to turn, do some deep soul searching.

Find Purpose, Direction, and Meaning - What do you love to do in your spare time? What ignites the passion in your heart and soul? Make a list of all the things you're good at and the things you love to do like: reading, writing, singing, dancing, painting, playing sports, or maybe playing a musical instrument. What kinds of things resonate deep within you?

Whistle While You Work - The things you love to do are directly related to your calling. It's about choosing a way of life that is consistent with your passions, desires, and personal gifts. Once you discover your life's purpose, try to find a way of making a living doing what you love, and working will never feel like work again.

64. Learn Something New Every Day

Make learning something new a part of your daily routine. Whether it's learning an interesting fact, or as challenging as learning a new language or musical instrument—the simple practice of learning deepens our character and makes us more confident.

We are All Learning Creatures - Surf the internet—type in something you've always wanted to know. Read, whether it's the morning newspaper, a magazine, a book, or whatever... Reading the newspaper keeps you up to date on what's going on in the world, and magazines usually contain all sorts of useful information on various topics. Watch educational television—the History channel, Animal Planet, and National Geographic. There is a lot of information on these channels.

Stay Interested and Interesting - By approaching life with a sense of curiosity, you keep yourself open to new experiences and opportunities. By staying interested and interesting, you'll be amazed how enriched and fulfilling your life can be.

65. Arouse & Nurture Your Passions

We all have a basic need to feel passionate about something. Whether it's about your relationships, music, hobbies, your job, your pet(s), or whatever else you feel deeply and strongly about... passion is a very powerful emotion. Passion is something that drives us emotionally. You know when you're passionate about something when you can't stop talking about it, or you get excited just thinking about it.

Ask Yourself Some Important Questions - It's important to nurture your passions from your heart and soul. What piques your interest? Is there something that you love to do? What sparks your creativity? Do you have a special hobby, or was there something you loved doing as a child?

Make a Bucket List - Coming from the term "kick the bucket," create a list of things you'd like to do before you die. Do you have a list of goals you'd like to achieve or any life-experiences or inner-passions you'd like to fulfill?

Express Your Passions - Most importantly, make sure you express passion for the things in life that truly matter —your kids, your spouse, your friends, and your pet(s). Sometimes we're so preoccupied with life in general, that we take our family and relationships for granted. Take the time to foster loving, trusting relationships. In the end, what's more important, knowing you gave and received love and made the most of your life, or sitting around with a big pile of meaningless stuff?

66. Step Out of Your Comfort Zone

Change can be scary. Your comfort zone is a comfortable place to be, because you know it's safe and predictable. On the other hand, your comfort zone may be limiting you to all sorts of life's possibilities. You could be missing out on love, financial opportunities, and a whole lot of fun. Yes, it's a little intimidating to take a risk, but sometimes we just need to face our fears and jump in. When you break free of your comfort zone, you're opening up your mind to new experiences.

Embrace Change - Exploring the unknown can be a frightening experience, but it can also bring you a world of passion, excitement, new friends, and new adventures. Without change, you may be missing out on some of life's greatest pleasures.

Don't Let Fear Control You - If fear of the unknown is holding you back from the life you truly desire—realize there are no guarantees in life. None of us know what is around the next corner. By overcoming fear of the unknown, we remove a huge mental obstacle, allowing us to develop as a person, while building a better life in the process. Overcoming something that terrifies us can truly be mentally liberating.

Where the Magic Happens - If you find you are paralyzed by fear of the unknown or uncertainty, just realize that the unknown may be a better, more positive place and may actually make you a happier, healthier person.

251

67. Adjust Your Attitude

Sometimes we are our own worst enemies. People often create chaos and stress in their lives through their own negative, self-defeatist, and worrisome attitudes. By simply adjusting our attitudes and realizing that we are in charge of how we react to any given situation, we can quite literally transform our lives. Many of our problems aren't caused by bad luck or other people, we create them within our own minds.

Stop Jumping to Conclusions - We've all been guilty of making assumptions or jumping to conclusions at one time or another. We develop an opinion about someone or something, before getting all the facts—and to make matters worse, we often times jump to conclusions in a negative way. But, if you think about it, this kind of thinking is irrational. We are not mind-readers or fortune tellers. Learn to bite your tongue, ask more questions, and weigh all the facts first. This will lead to fewer misunderstandings, less conflicts, and better relationships.

Stop Being Such a Perfectionist - Perfectionism is just an illusion. Nobody and nothing in life is perfect. Stop wasting precious time and energy trying to attain the unattainable. Just try to do your best, and be the best you can be. Imperfection can be a beautiful thing.

Let Go of the Past - For many of us, much of the anger, frustration, and misery we feel in our lives is directly correlated to past hurts or painful events that we can't let go of. Many people carry the past around with them like a big ball and chain, reliving and rehashing painful memories and heartache over and over again in their minds. When you obsess over the past, it festers, and slowly kills your spirit. Letting go of the past can free you to create the life you desire. Do not waste the short, precious time you have here on earth worrying about the things you cannot change.

Stop Sweating the Trivial Stuff - By learning to let go of the past and accepting the way things are, having realistic expectations, looking at the big picture, recognizing you do have a choice, and keeping a positive attitude— you will ultimately release the chains that bind you and you'll be able to open your heart to peace, happiness, and serenity. Learning to stop worrying about the things you have no control over, and instead learning to live with acceptance, is one of the most powerful gifts you can give to yourself and others. Make it a priority to embrace love, happiness, compassion, forgiveness, and gratitude. Changing your attitude can quite simply change your entire life.

68. Laugh Your Troubles Away

Laughing has a magical effect on the entire body. Laughing rejuvenates the mind, body, and spirit, and soul. The simple act of laughing causes a number of chemical changes in the body, triggering the release of the hormones, endorphins and serotonin. These hormones create the feelings of happiness, love, and euphoria.

Laughter is the Best Medicine - The positive physical, mental, and emotional effects of laughter are many. It improves mood, increases pleasure, reduces stress, strengthens the immune system, oxygenates the cells and internal organs, lowers blood pressure, suppresses pain both emotionally and physically, and aids in disease prevention. Laughing, exercising, and having an orgasm, are all excellent ways of raising your endorphin levels. If you're not having at least one good belly laugh a day, you're neglecting one of the most powerful anti-aging secrets of all!

Laugh Your Way to Wellness with Laughter Yoga - Do you want more joy and happiness in your life? Try the latest health craze sweeping the nation, "Laughter Yoga." Laughter Yoga is a fun, yet simple concept with a powerful impact which promotes physical, emotional, and mental well-being, while boosting your immune system and lowering stress.

Laughter Yoga - A Life Changing Experience - Laughter Yoga was created by physician and author, Dr. Madan Kataria. Together with his wife Madhuri, a yoga teacher, the first laughter yoga club was launched in Mumbai, India in 1995. Since then, it has become a worldwide phenomenon with over 8,000 laughter clubs in over 80 countries. This therapeutic laughter routine involves yogic breathing, laughter exercises, and stretching. It can be performed by people of all ages, and from all walks of life, and has been found to be a powerful antidote for those suffering from depression, as well as chronic illness.

The Many Health Benefits of Laughter:

Releases Endorphins - This "feel good" hormone lifts your spirits, giving you an optimistic attitude, self-confidence, and feelings of self-worth.

Strengthens Immune System - Laughter increases lymphatic flow which is proven to boost the immune system.

Oxygenates Organs - Laughter massages the internal organs which increases circulation, helping to flush the organs of toxins.

Anti-Aging - Laughter tones facial muscles which helps reduce fine lines and wrinkles, along with sagging skin. Just the simple act of laughing is shown to slow down the aging process.

69. Make Friends and Be Social

Socializing is extremely important, especially as we age. The act of socializing keeps us young at heart. Human-beings are social creatures, we all need companionship and to feel connected. Loneliness and social isolation can be very toxic and unhealthy, causing depression and loss of self-esteem, especially as we get older.

It's important to surround ourselves with friends and to have people in our lives to help support us and cheer us on through challenging times. We also need the camraderie and interaction of others to laugh with us when times are good. Having good friends and being around other people keeps us from feeling isolated and alone, and can make our lives richer and more fulfilling.

Become a Social Butterfly - Studies show, that people with many friends tend to outlive those with few friends. So, get out there, have fun, and socialize. Take a friend to lunch, go to a movie, host a party, travel with friends, attend church functions, or social events. Thanks to the latest technologies, it's now easier than ever to grow your circle of friends. Connect with old friends or classmates online or make new friendships with people with common interests.

Make Friendships a Priority - Social connections are vital to our physical and mental health and well-being. Socializing with friends and family lifts the spirits, improves cognitive skills, keeps the mind sharp, and helps prevent dementia.

70. Slow Down and Pay Attention

Our lives are more stressful and hectic than ever! With all this new modern technology that is supposed to be helping us save time, instead we're connected to our cell phones and laptops more than ever—checking text messages and emails, and no longer really focusing on what we're doing, as we're multi-tasking like crazy. When we spend time with family and friends, we're with them physically, but many times we're not really paying attention or fully listening, as we're distracted by our devices.

Remembering Life Before Cell Phones - It's hard to believe that not that awful long ago, life actually existed without cellphones. Whatever happened to the days when you could have a conversation without having to wait until someone sends off a 'quick text' or takes a call when you're in the midst of talking? And while cell phones sure do come in handy, especially in emergency situations, many people are becoming totally dependent on their phones and let phone calls or text messaging interfere with their daily lives and schedules.

Be a Good Listener - Interruptions and distractions are two of the biggest drains on our focus, energy, and productivity. Being in this state, can leave you overwhelmed, stressed-out, and dissatisfied with life in general. It's time to turn off our digital devices and make a conscious effort to be less distracted, while shifting our focus, and really paying attention to what really matters most—people we love, and who love us.

Reconnect WITHOUT Distractions - Slow down, take a deep breath, and really be mindful of what's going on around you. Live in the present moment, reconnect with yourself and others, and without distractions.

71. Think Positive Thoughts

Did you know that the average person has roughly 60,000 thoughts a day? Of these 60,000 thoughts, 95% are the same thoughts we had the day before, and the day before that. But even more surprising, is that for most of us, nearly 80% of these habitual and repetitive thoughts are negative.

Shift Your Thoughts and Change Your Life - The way you think, affects all aspects of your life. A positive attitude is not only a powerful antidote to aging, but makes it easier to deal with stress, worry, and negative thinking. Looking on the bright side lifts your endorphin levels, gives you more confidence, and enhances your health. Maintaining a positive attitude isn't always easy, but it is vital for overall health and can be a significant factor in bolstering the immune system to help fight off illness and disease, while giving you strength to get through times of stress.

It's All in Your Head - Changing your thoughts creates changes in the brain. By thinking optimistically, you not only change your brain chemistry, but you can actually increase your odds of living longer! It may not seem like it, but being optimistic is a choice you make, and it obviously doesn't come natural to everybody. It's something you have to work at from moment to moment.

Reprogram Your Thinking - If your negative attitude has become a perpetual habit, reprogram your thinking. Read self-help books, listen to motivational tapes, meditate, do EFT tapping, or recite daily affirmations or inspirational quotes.

Enjoy the Journey - Metaphorically, life is like a roller coaster ride—there's always going to be ups and downs —that's just part of the balance of life. It's just a matter of accepting that fact, focusing on the positive, and enjoying the journey! You have the power to choose if you want to be positive or negative, happy or unhappy. It's how you choose to react during the hard times that arise, that can help you make it through in one piece. Even eternal optimists have bad days, but an optimist chooses to look on the bright side—focusing on solutions, rather than problems—and opportunities, rather than hurdles.

Rx for Longevity - Studies show that people who are optimists and see the glass as half-full, rather than half-empty, are better able to handle stress, get sick less often, and experience more success in relationships, work, and all aspects of life. And one more reason to cop a positive attitude—having a positive attitude as you get older, can actually add 7 years to your life.

72. Keep the Focus On You

If you find yourself saying, "Stop the world, I want to get off!"... you are not the only one! Most of us women, and many men too, have at some time or another, found ourselves at the bottom of our to-do list when it comes to taking care of ourselves.

You Have to Look Out for #1 - YOU! It's not being self-centered, self-absorbed, or narcissistic! As women, we're so preoccupied with taking care of our husbands (or significant other), the kids, the housework, family finances, appointments, grocery shopping, and on and on —that often times we deny our own needs, and lose ourselves in the process.

Have Healthy Self Love - Learn to love yourself uncon- ditionally. If you don't feel good about yourself, you will continue to struggle with feeling successful in all areas of your life. By having healthy self-love and taking excellent care of yourself and your needs, you will be a happier, healthier, more productive person and will have more energy and optimism to give to others.

Own Your Power - Having healthy self love and self- compassion is about loving and accepting yourself just the way you are, and being true to who your are. It's about knowing your limitations and not saying yes, when you really mean no. You give away your power when you give in to what others want you to do, rather than what you want to do. Especially in situations when you let others negatively influence you, put you on a guilt trip, intimidate you, or control you. When you have healthy self-love and self-compassion, you do what's healthy for you, rather than what's harmful to you. Learn to accept yourself, and love yourself, and use that love to motivate healthy behavior.

Bottom Line: To truly become successful in life, at work, with family, and relationships, it's crucial to put taking care of ourselves at the top of the list, before we can tend to the needs of others.

73. Live in the Present Moment

We live in such a fast paced society that sometimes we get so busy, we forget to pay attention to what is going on around us. We spend so much of our time either thinking about past events, or planning for the future, that we miss out on what's happening in the present moment. Many of us live our lives on auto-pilot, not really paying attention, or being aware, and not really focusing on what we're doing, thinking, or feeling.

Life is really about all the little moments that happen every day. While we obsess or dwell over past or future events, life is passing us by. When you live with "consciousness" or "conscious living" you bring your focus and awareness into the present moment, and all worries of the past, and all fears of the future fade away.

Live Life Like There is No Tomorrow - Living in the present moment, and sometimes referred to as mindfulness, allows us to feel awake, alive, aware, and energized. If we live our lives with mindfulness, we will get so much more out of life. Stop and look around you. Use all your senses. Focus on the beauty that surrounds you. See the vibrancy of the colors of nature. Breathe in the air. Feel the sunshine on your face. Children live in the moment. Rediscover your inner-child.

So, How Do You Start Living in the Moment? Living in the moment is a process that takes practice. Yoga and meditation are both incredibly effective practices that teach you to quiet your mind and live more fully in the present moment. Also, if you go to the library, browse any book store, or surf the web, you will find an abundance of very insightful books and CD's/DVD's dedicated to teaching us how to start living our life in the "here and now," and achieving inner peace.

74. Let Go of Negative Emotions

You are the creator of your life. If you live with chaos and turmoil, you may find you're disorganized, your mind and surroundings are cluttered, and your life feels chaotic and overwhelming.

If you make poor choices, surround yourself with negative people and negative influences, and live a life filled with anger, contempt, and pessimism, then your life will reflect sheer negativity.

Negativity Causes Toxicity - Hate, jealousy, prejudice, worthlessness, cynicism, resentment, and greed are all negative emotions that accelerate the aging process. Negative emotions just drag you down and zap your energy, causing toxicity in the body and opening your door for sickness and disease. Replaying negative experiences over and over in your mind, only wedges it deeper into the brain.

Choose Positivity - On the other hand, if you choose to make intelligent choices, and surround yourself with people who are positive, encouraging, and supportive, chances are you will be more optimistic, self-confident, fulfilled, and successful in all areas of your life. Positive influences tend to cultivate more positive outcomes. Know that you have control over many things that happen to you. Your life reflects the thoughts that you project. Positive actions and feelings breed even more positivity.

Time to Say Goodbye - In addition to letting go of negative emotions, let go of people and things that drain your energy! Life is way too short to spend it with people who bring you down or doing things that make you unhappy! Surround yourself with people that lift your spirits and make you feel good about yourself.

Let Go of the Clutter - Each and every one of us has "stuff" that we've accumulated over the years. Some of our stuff, like prized possessions, have strong sentimental value, while other stuff is just basically clutter that we hold on to, but is really no longer useful to us. Even if you're emotionally attached, holding on to "piles of stuff" can make your life feel stagnant and overwhelming, while causing feelings of chaos and depression. Disencumbering yourself from useless clutter can be difficult at first, but in the long run, it can be extremely freeing, empowering, and energizing.

75. Treasure Life's Simple Pleasures

The key to happiness is NOT the ritzy house or fancy cars—it's being able to appreciate the simple pleasures and joys in life, like...

- Hugging your Child/Grandchild

- Listening to Up-Beat Music

- Watching Animals in Nature

- A Good Home-Cooked Meal

- The Smell of Fresh-Brewed Coffee

- Helping Someone in Need

- The Feeling After a Good Work-Out

- Watching a Beautiful Sunrise or Sunset

- A Good Wine

- The Beauty & Fragrance of Fresh Flowers

- Snuggling in Bed

- Fresh-Baked Chocolate Chip Cookies

- Getting a Relaxing Massage

- Taking a Hot Bath by Candlelight

- A Sensual Night With Your Partner

- Giving or Receiving a Compliment

- Catching Up With an Old Friend

- Singing in the Shower

- Witnessing a Double Rainbow

- Watching Humming Birds

- Walking Into a Clean House

- Laughing Till Your Sides Ache

- Looking Through a Kaleidoscope

- Gazing at the Stars

- Reminiscing About the Good Old Days

- Looking Through Old Photographs

- Dancing to Some Oldies But Goodies

- Finishing Your To-Do List

- Accomplishing Something You've Been Putting Off

The Possibilities are Endless!!!

76. Keep a Gratitude Journal

Keeping a gratitude journal is an extremely powerful way to retrain your thoughts and reduce negativity in your life, while helping you get into the habit of focusing your attention on the things in life for which you are thankful. By focusing on gratitude, we become more conscious and aware of the positive and good things in our lives.

Commit Yourself - Using something as simple as a spiral notebook, or as elaborate as a decorative journal—every night before bed, commit yourself to writing down 5 (or more) things that happened throughout the day (no matter how big or small) for which you are grateful. It may be something as simple as enjoying a decadent dessert or watching a beautiful sunset, or something huge like the birth of a child/grandchild or finishing a 5K race.

Express Gratitude - People who are grateful tend to be happier, healthier, less stressed, and more fulfilled. The simple act of expressing gratitude inspires us to recognize the simple things that normally we may have taken for granted or overlooked.

We Attract What We Think About - The Law of Attraction says that we attract what we think about, whether it be negative or positive. So, even on the days when you're feeling a little down, write in your gratitude journal and approach each and every day with an attitude of thankfulness.

77. Celebrate Life and Find Magic in Every Day

Living life to the fullest, celebrating life, and finding magic in everyday is a matter of creating balance in your life. It's about building loving relationships, learning to take control, learning from your mistakes, making the right choices, living with a positive attitude, maintaining good health & fitness, and achieving inner-peace and well-being.

Live Life With a Sense of Urgency - Everyone procrastinates, some worse than others. Maybe procrastinating is not that big a deal when it comes to unimportant, trivial issues—but when you're putting off things that will bring you happiness and fulfillment—that is a big deal! Visualize the kind of life you want—your dreams and desires—then set goals, take action, and go for it!

Life is Short - Eternity Isn't! It's time to celebrate getting older while learning to accentuate the positive. Savor every moment. Start celebrating the beauty, magic, and wonder of everyday life. Just remember, that this day you are currently living, will only happen once. How can you make the most of it?

Bottom Line: You are responsible for your life, no one else, and you alone have the power to change it. Learn to let go of stress, negativity, adversity, and disappointment and embrace the moment. Make a choice to seize the day and live life to the fullest. Love yourself, love what you do, and surround yourself with people that you love, and who love you.

In Review...

Study after study shows that no matter how old, or how sedentary and physically inactive you are, you can immediately begin to reverse the aging process. Millions of people suffer needlessly from illness and disease that could be prevented or reversed through healthy lifestyle changes. It's time to stop taking our health for granted and to take major strides towards better health and disease prevention. If longevity is your goal and you truly want to live a long healthy life—master the art of loving and respecting yourself enough to take excellent care of yourself inside and out.

Incorporating a healthy lifestyle isn't about making drastic changes—drastic changes are often times a recipe for failure. By making small, but consistent, healthy changes in your diet and lifestyle, you will begin to see numerous, positive changes in yourself. You'll find your mood will brighten, you'll feel less stressed, you'll have more energy, your eyes will sparkle, and your skin will glow with health.

NOTE: According to anti-aging experts, by incorporating healthy life-style choices into your daily life, you can begin to reverse the aging process and add many quality years to your life.

Healthy Lifestyle Choices That Can Add Years To Your Life:

Exercising on a regular basis and staying active (+4 years)

Practicing yoga, tai chi, or qigong (+4 years)

Practicing meditation regularly (+3 years)

Eating a fiber-rich diet (+2 years)

Consuming omega-3 fatty acids foods or supplements daily (+3 years)

Taking your vitamins and anti-aging supplements every day (+3 years)

Getting adequate sunshine and vitamin-D (+2 years)

Flossing daily and having healthy gums (+6 years)

Having at least one good belly laugh a day (+7 years)

Owning a pet (+5 years)

Keeping your brain healthy by doing activities that stimulate the mind (+4 years)

Having a strong social base and good friends (+7 years)

Being a happy person and having a positive/optimistic attitude (+7 years)

Having a healthy sex life (2-3 times a week) - (+4 years)

Unhealthy Lifestyle Choices That Can Subtract Years From Your Life:

Smoking cigarettes (-8 years)

Binge drinking (-4 years)

Suffering from chronic depression (-5 years)

Living with chronic stress (-4 years)

Having low self-esteem (-4 years)

Thinking old (-5 years)

Having bad genes (-10 years)

Being obese (-3 years)

Being morbidly obese (-10 years)

Eating an abundance of fast/junk food (-4 years)

Eating a high refined sugar diet (-4 years)

Having bad posture (-2 years)

Being an inactive couch potato (-8 years)

Not getting enough sleep (-5 years)

Having high blood pressure (-5 years)

Having diabetes (-7 years)

Having dementia (-5 years)

Now...

if you're feeling a little overwhelmed with all this information and you're wondering where do I begin my journey to
good health and longevity??

**Here are a Few Suggestions That Will Get You
Started on the Road to Healthy Aging and Youthful
Energy:**

Become More Aware - In order to change negative behavior and thought patterns, it's vital to become more
aware. If you're stuck in a rut and you don't know where
to start—start writing. For the next few days, or however
long you need, write down your thoughts, feelings, and
behaviors. Include everything you eat and drink, your
good and/or bad habits, your sources of stress, your
negative and positive actions, etc. Do your negative,
unhealthy thoughts and behaviors outnumber your posit-
ives? As human beings we all get stuck in habitual patterns. By being more conscious and aware, this is the
first step to becoming unstuck. Once you replace your
negative actions with healthy, positive ones—you will
start seeing powerful, life-changing results!

Breathe Deep, Stretch, and Let the Sunshine in - First
thing in the morning, take a few deep breaths and
stretch. Your body has been inactive for 7-9 hours and a
good stretch helps shake off sleepiness, awakens stiff
muscles, and gets the blood circulating. Then open the
blinds and let some sunlight in. Letting in natural light
takes the body out of sleep mode, energizes the body,
and stimulates the brain to stop producing the sleep hormone melatonin.

Exercise - A good morning workout triggers endorphins and lowers stress hormones, while giving you an energy boost that can last all day. Whether you take a brisk morning walk, or take a yoga class... a minimum of 30 minutes of cardio, 3-4 times a week, along with strength training, twice a week, will help rev up your energy levels, while building your endurance, stamina, and strength. **Refer to Tip #4.**

Drink Green Tea Instead of Coffee - Instead of your usual cup of coffee in the morning, try a hot cup of antioxidant rich green tea with a touch of manuka honey, for its many health and anti-inflammatory benefits. **Refer to Tip #28.**

Eat a Nutrient Rich Diet - Food is fuel for our body. Eating nutrient dense foods ensures you're getting the nutrition your body needs. Opt for a healthy diet of lean meats, poultry, fish, organically grown fruits and vegetables, fiber-rich whole grains, beans and legumes, nuts and seeds, and low fat dairy products. For optimal health, be sure each meal is nutritionally balanced, containing lean protein, complex carbohydrates, and healthy fats like extra virgin olive oil. **Refer to Tips #6, #11, & #12.**

Avoid Irregular Eating Patterns - Eating 5-6 small frequent meals throughout the day helps maintain a steady supply of nutrients to the body. It stabilizes blood sugar levels, keeps your metabolism stoked to help burn more calories, and gives you more energy and stamina. But eating more often isn't for everyone. If you have a problem with portion control or staying disciplined, just make sure you're not exceeding your daily calorie allotment and that you're making healthy food choices, and not skipping meals (especially breakfast). Start your day with a wholesome balanced breakfast such as whole grain cereal with fruit, eggs with whole grain toast, oatmeal, yogurt, or a healthy fruit smoothie.

Take an Anti-Aging Multi-Vitamin - Along with a healthy balanced diet, make sure to supply your body with all the nutrients it needs to function properly, by taking a good anti-aging multi-vitamin containing powerful and energizing cell rejuvenating antioxidants. Also, for those who do not eat fish or foods that contain omega-3 fatty acids—a 500 mg. supplement is recommended. For digestive health, take digestive enzymes during or immediately after each meal. **Refer to Tips #7 & #15.**

Avoid Processed Junk Food - Limit, or better yet, completely avoid foods with little or no nutritional value such as foods containing white flour, refined sugars, and high fructose corn syrup. Also, watch your intake of refined vegetable oils, artificial sweeteners, food additives, and foods high in sodium. Opt for healthy whole foods (food in its natural state) and preferably organic. **NOTE:** Health is not about deprivation. If you're a die hard sugar junkie, don't think you have to give up all your favorite sweet treats—just make sure you get in your healthy food choices first, and then enjoy your sweets in moderation. **Refer to Tips #6 & #14.**

Drink Plenty of Water - Lubricate your body by drinking plenty of water throughout the day, and especially first thing in the morning upon awakening. Water is essential for dehydration prevention, flushing out toxins and wastes, oxygenation of cells, healthy digestion, and decreasing the risk of many cancers. There is no substitute for water! **Refer to Tip #3.**

Take a Spiritual Break - The practice of daily meditation has numerous physiological, psychological, and spiritual health benefits and is a wonderful way to relieve stress and strengthen the body's immune system. **Refer to Tip #2.**

Practice Deep Breathing - Let your anxiety melt away by practicing deep breathing exercises every day. Deep breathing is a powerful relaxation technique that improves both physical and mental wellness by releasing tension from the body and clearing the mind. In addition, this simple exercise oxygenates every cell in the body and gives you boundless energy. **Refer to Tip #34.**

Soak Up Energy From the Sun - Take a walk, breathe in fresh air, and spend some time in nature. Our best source of vitamin-D is sun exposure. The sun helps alleviate depression and fatigue and is extremely energizing. Just 15-20 minutes of sunshine 3-4 days a week is enough to produce the body's requirement of vitamin-D. If you remain outside any longer than that, apply a natural sunscreen. **Refer to Tip #48.**

Keep Your Positive Energy Flowing - If you want to truly enhance your life and bring in a positive energy flow... stop thinking about what's wrong in your life, and start focusing on what's right. A positive attitude is very healing and energizing. A good place to start is with a gratitude journal. By keeping a gratitude journal you become more conscious and aware of the positive things in life that you are grateful for. **Refer to Tips #71 & #76.**

Get a Good Night's Sleep - Getting enough sleep is critical for proper brain function, keeping the heart healthy, reducing stress, and repairing the body. Sufficient sleep promotes good physical health, longevity, and emotional well-being. **Refer to Tip #9.**

In Conclusion...

There are many things in life that we can't control, but we are in control when it comes to how we treat our bodies—what we eat and drink, and the thoughts we think.

Like all life's journeys, changing your lifestyle begins with a single step... It's up to you. You just need to have the willingness and desire to begin the journey.

So... Take excellent care of yourself, think happy thoughts, and have fun exploring these powerful, natural, anti-aging, immune boosting tips for optimal health and longevity!

Here is a Quote That We All Need to Take Very Seriously...

"We don't catch diseases; we create them by breaking down the natural defenses according to the way we eat, drink, think, feel, and live."

"Herings Law of Cure," which is the basis of all healing.

And Last, But Not Least...

Are You Looking For Some Quick and Easy Budget-Friendly Beauty Tips??

Here are 30 Tried & True Beauty Tips, Anti-Aging Secrets, and Makeup Tricks for Healthy Glowing Skin, Shiny Hair, Kissable Lips, and More!

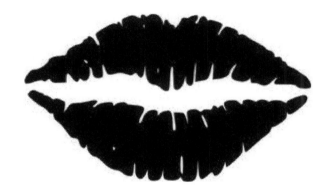

Part IX:

30 Outrageously Awesome Natural Beauty Tips

1. Brighten elbows by rubbing them with half a lemon. Lemons have a natural bleaching effect. Moisturize elbows afterwards to counteract the drying effects of the juice.

2. If you find it painful to tweeze eyebrows—hold an ice cube over the brow area first to numb the area. Using Baby Orajel also works well.

3. Brighten dark circles and tighten baggy puffy eyes with chilled raw potato slices, cucumber slices, or cooled wrung-out decaffeinated tea bags. Just place over the eyes and relax for 10-15 minutes.

4. Soak dry, brittle finger nails in a small bowl of warm extra-virgin olive oil (which is high in antioxidants) once a week to strengthen them and soften cuticles.

5. To stimulate eyelash growth—carefully coat your lashes with emu oil, olive oil, or castor oil using a Q-tip before going to bed, making sure not to get it into your eyes.

6. For dry skin on hands and feet—apply extra-virgin olive oil and put on gloves or white socks before going to bed. EVOO also works well for elbows and knees.

7. Keep your smile looking its best—make your own tooth whitening paste by adding 3 drops of hydrogen peroxide to 1 tablespoon of baking soda.

8. For beautiful skin—pour 2-3 beers into a warm bath and enjoy a beer bath. Beer is very good for the skin because it contains loads of vitamins, powerful antioxidants, and yeast.

9. For a quick pimple fix—apply a dab of toothpaste (DO NOT use gel) on the pimple and let it dry. The toothpaste may be left on for several minutes or overnight. Also, to calm a red, inflamed pimple, hold an ice cube over it for a few seconds to cool and soothe the skin.

10. Go very lightly with powder on fine lines and wrinkles around the eyes. Too much powder will settle into the wrinkles and actually emphasize them.

11. Run your freshly sharpened eyeliner pencil across a tissue before using it. This rounds off the sharp edges and removes any small particles or wood shavings.

12. To make your lips kissably soft—exfoliate dry chapped lips with a soft, wet toothbrush or washcloth. Gently rub in a circular motion to remove any flakiness and then apply lip balm.

13. To keep lipstick from getting on your teeth—once you've applied the lipstick, insert your index finger into your mouth and close your lips around your finger. Then slowly pull your finger out. The excess lipstick will come off on your finger.

14. Store skin care products and cosmetics in the refrigerator to extend the shelf-life and to minimize any health concerns caused by bacteria.

15. For overzealous eyebrow plucking—apply castor, coconut, or olive oil to your brows nightly before bed to stimulate growth, then wash off in the morning. Eyebrow regrowth is a slow process, so in the mean time, fill in any bald or sparse areas with an eyebrow pencil or eyebrow powder.

16. If you're prone to ingrown hairs—DO NOT shave in the opposite direction of hair growth. Instead, shave in the direction that hair grows, and use a moisturizing shave gel, or better yet, extra-virgin olive oil.

17. To fade stretch marks—dry brush every single day to exfoliate and stimulate blood circulation. Then rub a few drops of lavender, patchouli, or helichrysum essential oils mixed with good carrier oil such as sweet almond or jojoba into the stretch marks. These oils have regenerative effects that slow down aging of the skin, improve elasticity, and heal damaged skin cells.

18. To cure yellow finger nails caused by wearing dark-colored nail polish—rub with lemon juice, then rinse and massage hands and nails with a moisturizer.

19. To protect your skin from the harsh chemicals and to prevent hair-coloring from dying your skin, rub vaseline along your hairline.

20. If after using a self-tanner, you end up with streaks or blotchiness—put some baking soda on a wet loofah or washcloth and gently scrub in a circular motion. This works especially well for stained, callused feet, elbows, knees, or palms of the hands. **NOTE:** It's important to exfoliate the skin BEFORE applying a self-tanner for best results!

21. To get rid of dandruff—add a few drops of aromatherapy essential oils like tea tree or eucalyptus to your shampoo.

22. To lighten and brighten your complexion—mix 1 part apple cider vinegar, 1 part lemon juice, and 1 part water. Soak a cotton ball in the solution, squeezing out excess, and rub over your face in the morning and again in the evening. This works well for melasma, age spots, and freckles.

23. For rock hard nails—add fresh, finely chopped garlic to a bottle of clear nail polish and let it sit for 7 days. The garlic hardens and strengthens the nails, so they are less likely to peel or break.

24. An inexpensive way to boost the shine of brunette hair is to rinse after shampooing with diluted apple cider vinegar. Blondes benefits from lemon juice applied the same way. Both act by sealing the outer cuticles of the hair, which helps to reflect the light.

25. Cover spider veins with a light covering of concealer, applied with a makeup brush, and set with a dusting of powder.

26. Rub a dab of vaseline around the neck of a new bottle of nail polish, and it should be easy to open for the life of the product.

27. To bring out your eye color—avoid matching your eye shadow to the color of your eyes. Use complimentary colors instead. **NOTE:** To remove eye makeup—extra-virgin olive oil is a simple solution. Just a drop or two on a cotton ball is all you need to gently and effectively remove eye makeup.

28. For whiter teeth—if your teeth have a grayish tone, use a warm-shade lipstick like bronze or copper. If your teeth are more yellow, pick cool blue-based lipstick shades.

29. To make your eyes sparkle and appear bigger—try outlining them just inside the upper and lower lashes with a soft white cosmetic pencil.

30. For bad breath—FLOSS! Flossing is a crucial step for dislodging food and bad breath bacteria that may linger. Daily flossing can add 6+ years to your life by removing bacteria which can cause inflammation and lead to heart disease. **NOTE:** For gum irritation and canker sores, mix 4 drops of myrhh essential oil with 4 oz. of water and swoosh around in your mouth. Repeat twice daily.

As you can see, there are so many simple, yet powerful steps you can take to help reverse aging and prolong your life, while significantly enhancing your health and appearance. I hope you've enjoyed my anti-aging, health, and beauty tips, and that you find the information helpful and inspritational in addressing your own anti-aging, skin care, and health and wellness concerns!

Live Well. Be Happy. Be You.

Here's to Living a Long, Happy, Healthy Life!

~Amy~

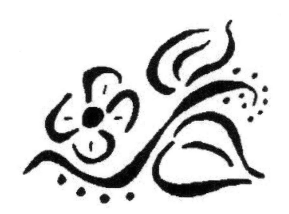